ALSO BY JULES ARON

Zen and Tonic: Savory and Fresh Cocktails for the Enlightened Drinker

Vegan Cheese: Simple, Delicious, Plant-Based Recipes

Nourish & Glow: Naturally Beautifying Foods & Elixirs

FRESH
&
PURE

FRESH & PURE

Organically Crafted Beauty Balms & Cleansers

Jules Aron

THE COUNTRYMAN PRESS
A division of W. W. Norton & Company
Independent Publishers Since 1923

For information about permission to reproduce selections from this book,
write to Permissions, The Countryman Press, 500 Fifth Avenue, New York, NY 10110

For information about special discounts for bulk purchases, please contact
W. W. Norton Special Sales at specialsales@wwnorton.com or 800-233-4830

Manufacturing by ToppanLeeFung
Production manager: Devon Zahn

The Countryman Press
www.countrymanpress.com

A division of W. W. Norton & Company, Inc.
500 Fifth Avenue, New York, NY 10110
www.wwnorton.com

978-1-68268-102-2

10 9 8 7 6 5 4 3 2 1

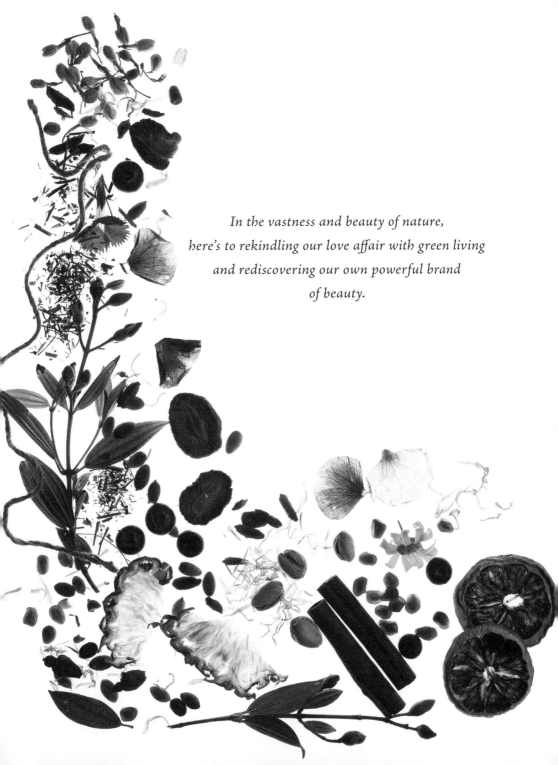

In the vastness and beauty of nature,
here's to rekindling our love affair with green living
and rediscovering our own powerful brand
of beauty.

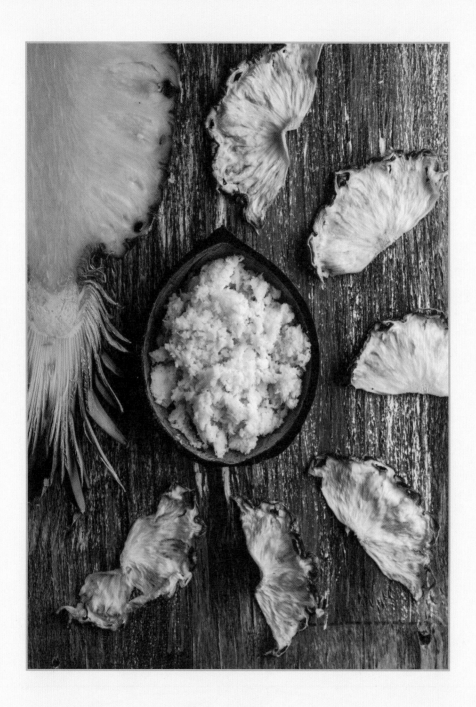

CONTENTS

Introduction 9

Natural Beauty Apothecary 13

Facial Skin Care 21

Natural Makeup 73

Body Care 89

Hand and Foot Care 135

Hair Care 147

Health and Hygiene 165

Spa Day Treats 177

Basic Apothecary Techniques 207

Resources and Further Reading 211

Acknowledgments 215

Index 217

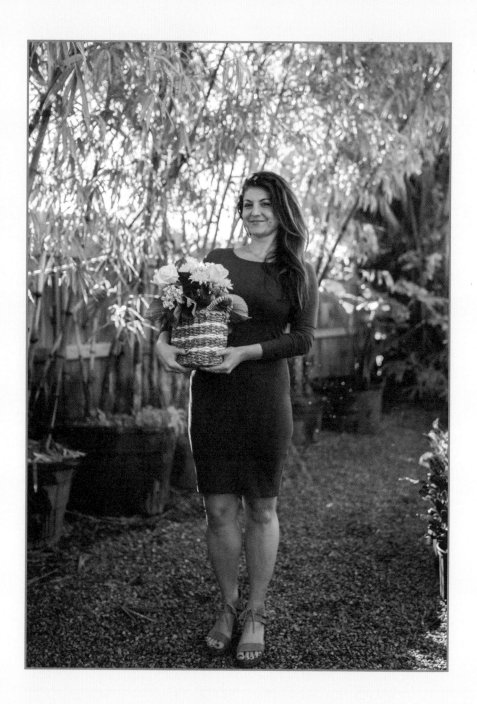

INTRODUCTION

Living in a modern world, with state-of-the-art technological advancements promising youth and beauty with every jar, treatment, or injection, it is easy to understand how we've moved so far away from simple holistic herbal practices.

But it is also easy to see that we feel better when we rely on real food, spend lots of time outdoors, and bring elements of nature into our daily lives. Our plant world has bestowed on us an incredible array of fruits, herbs, seeds, and flowers that have been used for generations for improved authentic beauty and well-being. Whole foods and botanicals are nourishing, pampering, cleansing, and balancing.

In *Fresh & Pure*, we'll nourish our skin with the same loving care we use to prepare our meals in *Nourish & Glow*. Together we'll explore holistic self-care rituals and rediscover natural beauty products for a beautiful, vibrant body and soul.

Embrace the ideas on these pages and have fun rediscovering your true beauty with simple, wholesome body care recipes and the many wellness inspirations peppered throughout this book. May this collection help us rethink our routines, seek out better habits, refresh our outlooks, and reconnect with nature and our true beautiful selves.

SKIN DEEP

Our skin is a living system that includes the hair, nails, glands, and receptors. It performs nine essential functions for our body:

+ Excretes salt, water, and toxins through sweat

+ Protects from physical, chemical, and biological damage

+ Regulates moisture

+ Responds to heat, cold, pain, and pleasure

+ Helps maintain a steady temperature

+ Prevents mineral loss

+ Converts sun rays into vitamin D_3

+ Metabolizes fat

+ Secretes sebum

It is also the largest organ of the body, capable of absorbing topical products directly into the bloodstream.

The truth is, many of the ingredients in commercial beauty products just aren't that pretty. With weak regulations and the FDA's limited role, personal care products are laden with industrial chemicals, including carcinogens, pesticides, reproductive toxins, and hormone disruptors.

We have been led to believe that the more it foams, the more it cleans; the more slippery it feels, the more hydrating it must be; the more we lather on, the more effective it will be. Yet cheap and easy ingredients, such as alcohol, sodium laureth sulfate, and mineral oil, which give us the sensation of being clean and moisturized, are the very same ingredients that slow the skin's ability to create healthy cells and strip it of its natural moisture.

It is time to take back our glow.

By returning to nature and simplifying our beauty routine, we can begin to make better choices.

THE PRETTY ZEN PHILOSOPHY

The Pretty Zen philosophy is deeply rooted in finding, balancing, and maintaining wholesome beauty in a modern world. Part philosophy, part lifestyle, Pretty Zen takes natural healing modalities, Eastern philosophies, integrative nutrition, and an overall holistic approach to well-being and applies them to a modern way of life. It is a natural outlook with an underlying belief that there may be no greater pursuit than a life well loved.

The following beauty lifestyle elements are at the core of the Pretty Zen philosophy. Incorporating these in the form of personal wellness practices will nurture your lasting beauty.

PILLARS OF A BEAUTIFUL LIFE

NUTRITION AND HYDRATION

Satisfying our daily nutrition and hydration needs is essential for our beauty and health. It is important to discover our own individual dietary needs. For recipe inspiration and more on essential nutritional needs, please pick up *Nourish & Glow,* the sister book to this one.

MOVEMENT

Our bodies thrive on movement, yet we all require different types of exercise and these needs may change over time. It's simply a matter of finding the right option for you. Stay open-minded and you'll find a routine that will nourish you on a regular basis.

SLEEP

When it comes to your beauty routine, sleep may be the closest thing to a fountain of youth. Your body repairs and recovers while you rest, and that leads to a long list of glow-getting benefits.

RELATIONSHIPS

The quality of our relationships greatly influences the quality of our lives. It is important to cultivate healthy, loving relationships that support our individual needs, wants, and desires.

MEDITATION AND MINDFULNESS

There is something very nourishing about feeling deeply connected: feeling the vastness when looking up at the sky, the sense of the infinite when sitting by the ocean, and taking the time to reconnect with our natural surroundings can all bring us great peace and nurture our well-being.

NATURAL BEAUTY APOTHECARY

Armed with a well-stocked beauty apothecary and a few simple techniques, you're ready to elevate your beauty care regimen to glowing proportions.

NATURAL INGREDIENTS

ALOE VERA: Anti-inflammatory, antibacterial, antiviral, moisturizing, and soothing. Reach for aloe vera gel's cooling effects when you have a sunburn or an itchy scalp.

AVOCADOS: Avocados' omega-3 and omega-9 fatty acids hydrate and moisturize the skin while their plant nutrients, minerals, and vitamins work to repair existing damage.

BAKING SODA: Add to your bath to ease sunburn, itching, or inflammation.

CASTILE SOAP: Plant-derived, mild biodegradable soap used as a base in shampoos, body washes, and household cleaners.

CLAY: Rich in minerals, clays are known for their ability to draw out oils, toxins, and impurities. Used in masks and scrubs, they also tighten and tone skin.

COCOA BUTTER: With an enchanting chocolate scent and vitamin E content, cocoa butter improves skin elasticity and stimulates collagen production.

ESSENTIAL OILS: Essential oils are the concentrated vital essences of aromatic plants. These botanical distillations with healing properties penetrate pores deeply to nurture skin from the inside out. (For more about essentials oils, see pages 108–109.)

LEMONS: Astringent, disinfecting, and stimulating, lemon juice works to purge waste from your cells.

MAPLE SYRUP: A natural humectant, maple syrup draws moisture from the air into the skin and ensures its retention in the layers where it's needed most for penetrating, long-lasting hydration.

Maple syrup is especially high in skin-loving minerals, such as calcium, iron, magnesium, phosphorus, sodium, potassium, and zinc.

OATS: Anti-inflammatory and antioxidant-rich oats promote healing and skin hydration. When used in cleansers, oats' natural saponins exfoliate skin and draw out toxins.

RAW APPLE CIDER VINEGAR: Antimicrobial, antibacterial, antiseptic, and pH balancing. The natural alpha hydroxy acids in raw apple cider vinegar work together to give your face a glow, enriching it with its enzymes, proteins, and good bacteria.

SEA SALT: Naturally high in minerals, sea salt is a natural disinfectant and an ideal exfoliant. Use in your bath water or in scrubs to allow your body to absorb minerals, such as magnesium, potassium, calcium, and sodium, through your epidermis.

SHEA BUTTER: Silky in texture, deeply nurturing, and easily absorbed by the skin, shea butter helps restore skin's elasticity due to its vitamin A and E content.

VEGETABLE WAX: Healing and moisturizing, wax is a natural preservative and emulsifier used to thicken balms and salves to add a protective barrier that seals nourishing moisture in.

WITCH HAZEL: The liquid extract of the witch hazel shrub, witch hazel is a skin-healing astringent loaded in antioxidants that soothes and calms irritated skin. Look for pure witch hazel that isn't diluted with alcohol.

BASE OILS

You'll also find yourself using base oils. These vegetable oils, made from the seed, nuts, or kernels of plants and filled with essential fatty acids, easily penetrate into the skin, facilitating the absorption through the skin of essential oils and herbal extracts when mixed into it.

Here are some common oils and their properties, to help you choose the best one for your needs:

ALMOND OIL: Protein-rich almond oil retains moisture, calms skin, and removes impurities. Its nourishing properties make it an ideal choice for an allover body moisturizer or massage oil.

APRICOT KERNEL OIL: A light oil that contains fatty acids and vitamin A, apricot oil is moisturizing, nourishing, and anti-inflammatory.

ARGAN OIL: Hydrating argan oil protects skin and dissolves excess sebum, making it an ideal choice for both hair and skin care.

AVOCADO OIL: Nutrient-rich avocado oil improves skin elasticity and increases collagen, making it a great option for facial care.

CASTOR OIL: Highly viscous, castor oil contains vitamin E, proteins, omega-6, and omega-9 that collectively heal damaged, inflamed skin. Castor oil is also known for its antibacterial properties and various medicinal benefits that can help restore skin's natural moisture and improve hair growth.

COCONUT OIL: Full of antioxidants and with antimicrobial and antifungal properties, coconut oil is an easily sourced choice for body and hair care.

GRAPESEED OIL: Extracted from the seeds of grapes, grapeseed oil is loaded with powerful antioxidants and natural plant compounds called oligomeric proanthocyanidin complexes, or OPCs, known for their potent antioxidant activity. Penetrating and slightly astringent, grapeseed oil can help restore collagen at the cellular level and offers antiseptic properties that can help reduce swelling and speed wound healing.

JOJOBA OIL: Jojoba is a light and quickly penetrating oil that mimics the action of sebum, the skin's own natural lubricant, making it an ideal facial oil that nourishes and protects the skin.

MACADAMIA OIL: Another excellent facial oil, macadamia oil is rich in palmitoleic acid, which is regenerative, astringent, and soothing and promotes young-looking, soft, and supple skin.

NEEM OIL: A traditional Ayurvedic oil, neem oil extract has medicinal properties, with antibacterial, antifungal, analgesic, and anti-inflammatory benefits. Neem oil can help condition the skin and reduce redness, swelling, itching, and pain, as well as prevent skin infections.

OLIVE OIL: Olive oil is packed with antiaging antioxidants and hydrating squalene, making it superb choice for hair, skin, and nails. Although it has a strong odor, olive oil is a simple, easy-to-find moisturizing ingredient.

ROSE HIP OIL: A powerful skin cell regenerator, rose hip oil can help prevent premature skin aging. It also contains vitamins C and E, giving it anti-inflammatory properties for skin conditions such as eczema and psoriasis.

VEGETABLE GLYCERIN: Naturally derived from plants, vegetable glycerin is a soothing skin emollient, lubricant, and humectant. Glycerin helps the skin retain its moisture and restore natural pH balance.

VITAMIN E OIL: Antioxidant-rich vitamin E is an excellent natural preservative that can be added to oil blends and salves to prolong their shelf life. Also beneficial on its own for soothing scars and stretch marks.

WHEAT GERM OIL: This nourishing oil is a great choice of oil for dry, mature skin. Its anti-inflammatory properties are also appropriate for the pain and swelling of eczema and psoriasis.

NATURAL BEAUTY TOOL KIT

Most of the tools you need to custom-make your beauty balms and cleansers are likely to be in your kitchen already.

Here is a list of basic tools to have on hand:

BLENDER OR FOOD PROCESSOR: You'll need this household appliance for whipping up lotions, creams, and body butters.

COFFEE OR NUT GRINDER: Perfect for pulverizing nuts, seeds, oats, and herbs into fine powders. A mortar and pestle will work, too.

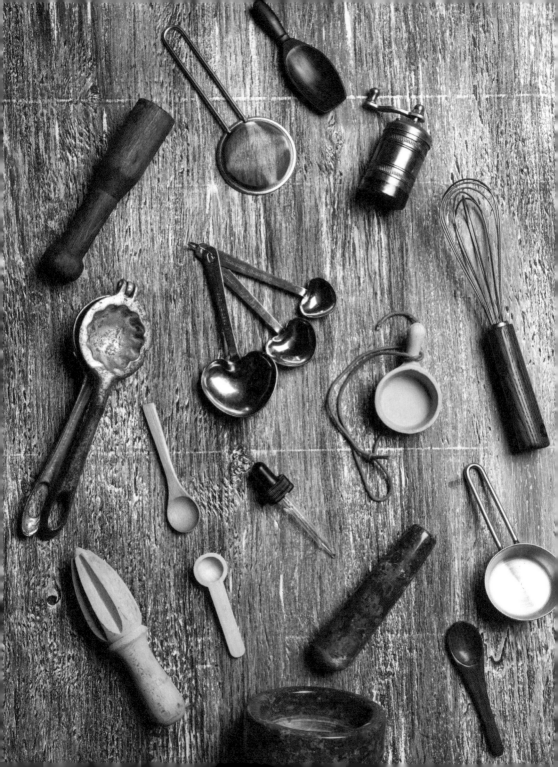

EYEDROPPERS: If you plan on adding essential oils to your beauty recipes, a pipette or an eyedropper is very useful to have on hand.

FINE-MESH STRAINER OR CHEESECLOTH: You'll need a strainer or cheesecloth to filter your beauty infusions.

FUNNEL: A small funnel will make pouring liquid ingredients into smaller bottles a breeze.

GLASS JARS: Small and large mason jars or amber glass jars make perfect containers to store your beauty recipes.

MEASURING CUPS AND SPOONS: Dedicate an inexpensive set of measuring spoons and glass measuring cups to your beauty recipes.

MIXING BOWLS: Glass mixing bowls in different sizes are useful to have on hand.

As you page through this book, resolve to make your daily moments of self-care into lasting beauty. The following collection of beauty-boosting recipes and self-care rituals create a solid foundation that will support your beautiful, well-nourished life.

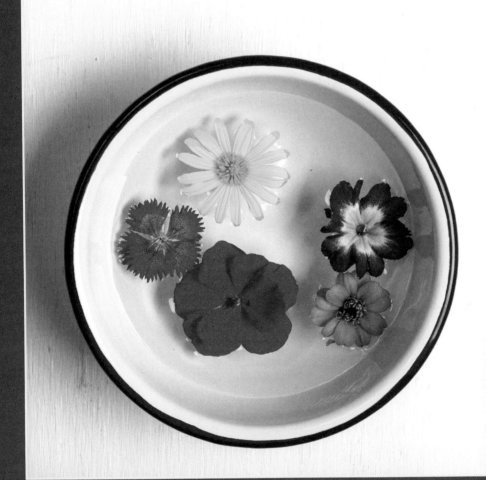

FACIAL SKIN CARE

Developing a beauty regimen is about feeling good in your skin and making self-care a priority.

Hibiscus Rejuvenating Cleansing Face Oil

Blueberry and Lavender Face Cleanser

Matcha Cleansing Grains

Deep Pore Treatment

Facial Steam pH Balancer

Pomegranate and Rose Hip Whipped Moisturizer

Rose Oil Elixir

Vitamin C Love Serum

Acai Berry Facial Mask

Sea Siren Mask

Beauty Carrot Mask

Papaya Face Scrub

Piña Colada Face Polish

Strawberries and Cream Face Polish

Apple and Green Tea Face Toner

Grapefruit Vanilla Face Mist

Cucumber Mint Aloe Face Wipes

Neck-Smoothing Compress

Nourishing Eye Balm

Cooling Eye Gel

Lash Serum

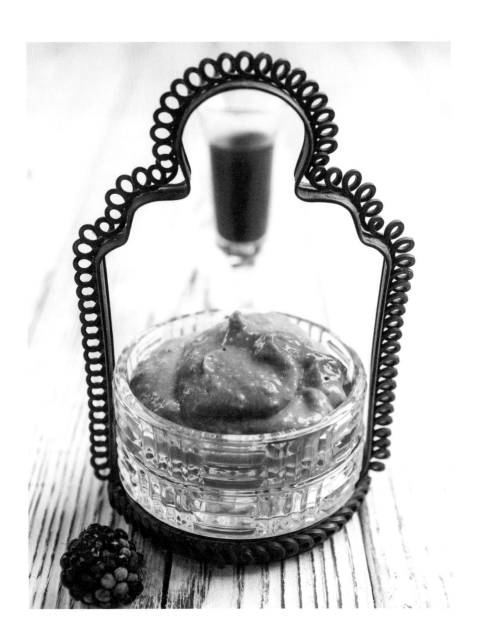

Gentle Ways to Come Clean

There's no better way to start and end the day than by cleansing your face of dirt and makeup residue. The issue with most commercial cleansers, however, is that they tend to strip the natural lipid layer from the skin's surface and destroy its protective barrier, leaving your skin feeling dry or tight.

The following three cleansing methods are gentle and effective substitutes for the harsh commercial varieties. Try them all before deciding on your preferred method.

DIY FACIAL AT HOME

Experts recommend that we get a facial every 4 to 6 weeks, but that can be hard to work into our budget. Here is a simple DIY facial routine you can effectively do at home.

CLEANSE: Remove all makeup and wash your face, neck, and ears, using your preferred facial cleanser from pages 26–35. Cleansing removes dirt, oil, and makeup to give your skin a clean slate. This allows all other products to penetrate optimally into the deeper layers of the skin.

Start by rinsing your face with lukewarm water. Then, using your middle and ring fingers, apply your choice of cleanser in circular motions. Rinse with lukewarm water and gently pat your skin dry with a washcloth.

EXFOLIATE: Using your fingers, gently rub your choice of facial scrubs from pages 52–56 in small circular motions all over your face. Make sure you focus on areas around your nose and forehead. If certain areas of your face are oilier than others, give that section an extra scrub. This would be a great time to do a lip scrub (see page 76).

STEAM: Steam is the most relaxing and cleansing part of a facial. There are a few ways to steam your face (I describe the process on page 36). For a quicker version, fill your sink with hot water, add some essential oils, and soak a washcloth in it. Wring out the washcloth and press it to your face. Breathe deeply. Repeat this step three times.

Get creative with your steam—add rose petals, rosemary, thyme, or any other favorite herbs.

MASK: After all of that deep cleaning, it's time for some pampering. The mask is the heart of any facial. It is when your skin is most ready to receive healing nutrients. Apply any of the face masks on pages 46–51 and leave it on for 15 to 20 minutes.

This would be a good time to try the Cooling Eye Gel (page 70), and don't forget the cucumber slices over your eyes! Breathe deeply and relax.

To remove, use a warm, damp washcloth. Finish with a splash of cold water.

MOISTURIZE: Now choose your favorite facial moisturizer (see pages 38–43) and massage your face deeply for 3 minutes. A facial massage is a great way to tone and lift the skin, and allow the healing oils to penetrate more deeply. Follow my steps for a DIY facial massage (pages 44–45). Finish with a spritz of your preferred toner or face mist (pages 59–60), or your favorite flower hydrosol.

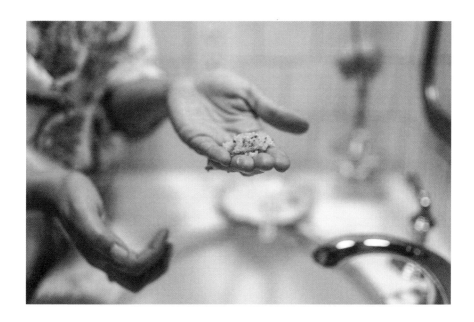

HIBISCUS REJUVENATING CLEANSING FACE OIL

The basic concept of cleansing with oil might seem counterproductive; however, following one of the most basic principles of chemistry, "Like dissolves like," the best way to dissolve a solvent, such as oil, is—you guessed it—by using another oil.

By using the right oils, you can cleanse your pores of dirt and bacteria naturally, gently, and effectively, while replacing the dirty oil with beneficial oils extracted from natural botanicals, vegetables, and fruit that heal, protect, and nourish your skin.

One of my absolute favorite oil infusions is made with the lovely hibiscus blossom. Not just a pretty flower, the hibiscus has been used in Ayurvedic and traditional Chinese medicine for its healing properties for centuries.

Recently coined the "Botox plant," hibiscus is a natural source of alpha hydroxy acids (AHAs), which can help speed up cell rejuvenation, control breakouts, and improve the elasticity of our skin.

With the addition of rose hip oil, rich in vitamin C antioxidants, this potent, synergistic blend also stimulates collagen production.

MAKES 3 OUNCES

¼ cup hibiscus-infused almond oil
1 teaspoon rose hip oil
1 teaspoon or 2 capsules vitamin E oil
10 drops bergamot essential oil (optional)

Mix together the oils in a small bowl and transfer to a lidded glass jar.

To use: Apply to your face and massage a small amount into your skin for 2 minutes. Place a warm, damp muslin cloth or washcloth over your face for an additional minute. Then gently rinse with warm water.

Store in its sealed glass jar in a cool, dry place. For maximum freshness and potency, please use within 6 months.

Best Oils for Your Skin Type

Want to experiment with your own oil blends? Follow these guidelines to find the best oil for your skin.

FOR OILY SKIN: *Choose oils with a high percentage of linoleic acid, which helps reduce blemishes by protecting your skin's surface. Try safflower, evening primrose, sunflower, or grapeseed oil, which can help regulate your natural oil production.*

FOR DRY SKIN: *Choose oils rich in fatty acids and polyphenols that are nourishing and help fight aging. Try macadamia, wheat germ, avocado, or neem oil.*

FOR NORMAL/COMBINATION SKIN: *Choose oils that have a percent ratio close to 50 percent of oleic acids and are more balanced for combination skin types without being too far on either side of the spectrum. Try almond, sesame, argan, apricot kernel, or rose hip oil.*

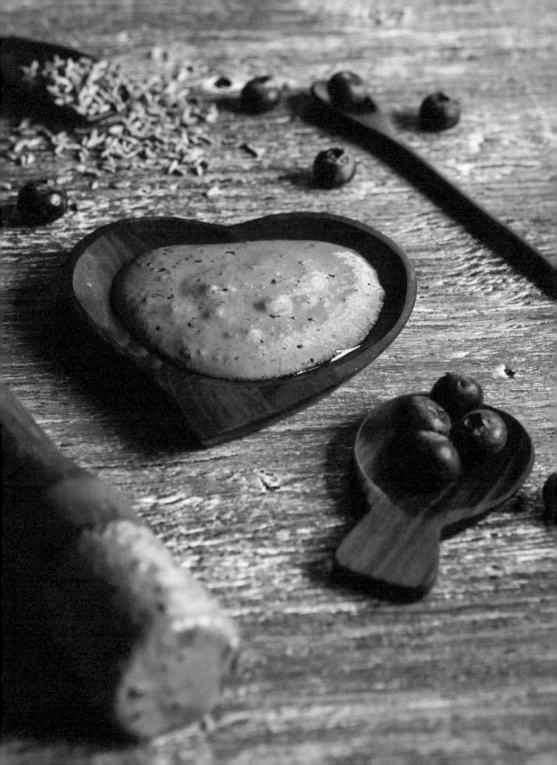

BLUEBERRY AND LAVENDER FACE CLEANSER

If you're not ready to jump into oil-based cleansers, this heavenly scented cleanser with witch hazel is a good option to start with. A plant-based substance with a long history of use for calming skin conditions, witch hazel adds a mild astringent quality to your facial cleansing ritual.

Top it off with vitamin- and antioxidant-rich blueberries—which boost collagen production—and you've got the recipe for healthy, glowing skin.

MAKES 3 OUNCES

10 blueberries
2 tablespoons almond oil
3 tablespoons witch hazel
10 drops lavender oil (optional)

Place all the ingredients in a blender and blend until smooth. Transfer to a lidded glass jar.

To use: Apply to your face and massage into your skin for 2 minutes, then rinse with warm water.

Store in its sealed glass jar in the refrigerator. For maximum freshness and potency, please use within 1 week.

✦ ✦ ✦ ✦

APOTHECARY TIP

When purchasing witch hazel, make sure to choose a brand that hasn't been distilled with alcohol. The alcohol-based versions can be drying to the skin.

✦ ✦ ✦ ✦

MATCHA CLEANSING GRAINS

The exceptional antioxidant properties of matcha tea and the detoxifying properties of clay work in harmony to nourish and rejuvenate cells and tissues at the deepest level, while absorbing dirt and impurities.

MAKES ⅓ CUP

1 tablespoon rolled oats
1 tablespoon flaxseeds
1 tablespoon almonds
2 tablespoons matcha powder
½ cup kaolin clay
5 drops chamomile essential oil (optional)

Combine the oats, flaxseeds, and almonds in a coffee grinder. Grind to a fine powder. Sift the dry mixture through a fine-mesh strainer into a glass, wooden, or ceramic bowl.

Add the matcha powder, clay, and essential oil, if using, and mix well, using a nonmetal spoon or spatula. Transfer to a lidded glass jar.

To use: Pour 1 tablespoon of the dry cleansing grains into the palm of your hand and mix with a few drops of water to create a paste. Apply to your face and massage into your skin, using circular motions. Leave the cleanser on your face for a few minutes to work its magic, then rinse with warm water.

Store in its sealed glass jar in a cool, dry place. For maximum freshness and potency, please use within 3 months.

✦ ✦ ✦ ✦

APOTHECARY TIP

To elevate your experience further, try using warm green tea instead of water to mix your cleansing grains, for an extra dose of antioxidants.

✦ ✦ ✦ ✦

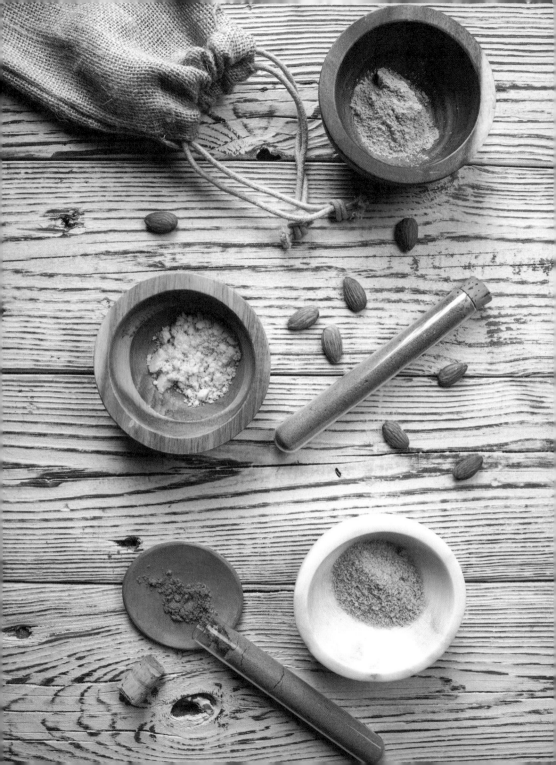

Why Clay?

The beautifying and purifying properties of clay have been used for thousands of years by cultures all around the world. Because of its molecular charge, clay naturally seeks out toxins on and in the body to bind with. Clay is also rich in beautifying minerals, including calcium, magnesium, silica, sodium, copper, iron, and potassium. Different clays have unique properties.

✦ ✦ ✦ ✦

APOTHECARY TIP

Clays are easily found in beauty supply stores, natural food co-ops, and online shops. Make sure to check the resource section at the end of the book. Do not use metal bowls or utensils when using clay. Clay absorbs and purifies toxins in the body because it is negatively charged. Touching metal, which is positively charged, deactivates some of clay's amazing benefits.

✦ ✦ ✦ ✦

WHICH CLAY IS RIGHT FOR YOU?

KAOLIN CLAY, OR WHITE COSMETIC CLAY: One of the most common and versatile clays used in cosmetic applications. White kaolin clay can be used in body powders, deodorants, face masks, and dry shampoos. It is also the perfect choice for sensitive skin.

RHASSOUL CLAY: This clay, mostly mined from the Atlas Mountains in Morocco, contains higher percentages of silica, magnesium, potassium, and calcium than other clays. Considered one of the most luxurious clays, rhassoul clay is often used in the most high-end spas around the world and works well for all skin types.

BENTONITE CLAY: High in bone-feeding minerals, such as calcium and potassium, bentonite clay is used in facial, body, and hair masks. It is even safe enough to take internally for detoxifying purposes. The mineral content in this clay also helps to remineralize the teeth. Bentonite clay is also great for all skin types.

FRENCH GREEN CLAY: This clay is not only high in minerals but also in decomposed plant matter that nourishes and remineralizes skin. Used extensively for its superabsorbent powers, French green clay is great for use on acne and oily skin types, helping to tighten pores and soak up excess sebum and oils.

FULLER'S EARTH: This clay, which comes from ancient volcanic ash sediments, makes a great oil absorber. It also has lightening and brightening properties, making it a good choice for evening skin tone and diminishing redness.

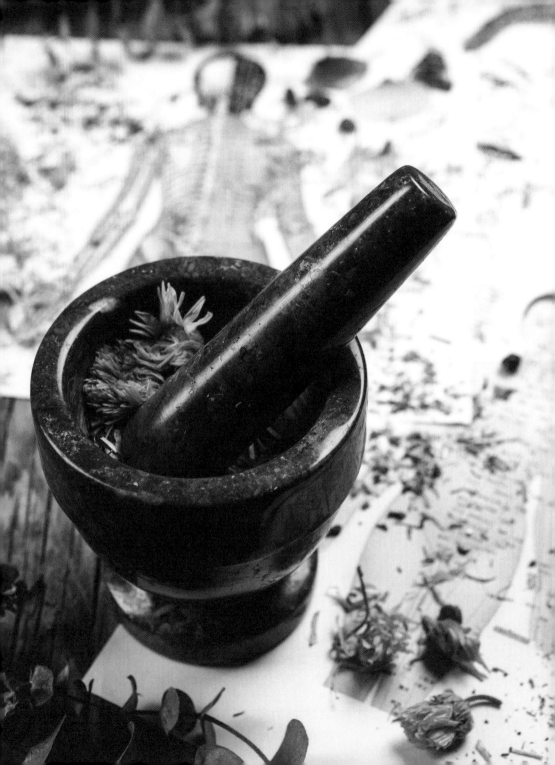

DEEP PORE TREATMENT

This penetrating oil treatment dissolves the impurities lodged deep in your pores. The steam opens your pores, allowing the oil to be removed gently and effectively.

MAKES 1 TREATMENT

2 tablespoons castor oil

To use: With your fingertips, gently apply the oil to your skin. Massage it into your face for 2 minutes.

Pass a washcloth under hot water, wring it out, and place it over your face. Allow the steam to penetrate your skin for a deep cleansing experience. Rinse your washcloth and repeat the process. Finally, use the damp washcloth to remove any oily residue.

✦ ✦ ✦ ✦

APOTHECARY TIP

There is some controversy over the harvesting and manufacturing practices of castor oil that expose workers to a compound that can be toxic. The finished castor oil is not toxic, however. But for those who prefer not to use castor oil due to its unsustainable growing practices, hazelnut, sunflower, or coconut oil also works wonderfully in its place.

✦ ✦ ✦ ✦

FACIAL STEAM pH BALANCER

Herbal facial steams are essentially teas for your face.

The warm, moist heat encourages the pores to open up, take a deep breath, and let vital moisture deep into the skins layers. Heat also brings oxygenated blood to the surface of your skin, at which point your facial tissues are gently prodded to release toxins, while the herbs release their oils, penetrating deep into your skin to promote healing.

MAKES 1 TREATMENT

1 tablespoon fresh chamomile
1 tablespoon fresh sagee
1 tablespoon fresh thyme
3 cups distilled water
¼ cup raw apple cider vinegar
Essential oils (optional)

Place the herbs in a piece of cheesecloth and tie into a bundle. Combine the distilled water and vinegar in a large pot and bring to a boil. Remove from the heat. Quickly add your herbal bundle to the hot liquid, cover, and let steep for 15 minutes. Add essential oils, if desired.

Place the pot on a solid, heatproof surface and drape a large bath towel over your head and the steaming pot. Close your eyes and breathe deeply, making sure to keep your face about 10 inches away from the pot. Finish the treatment by splashing cool water or a flower hydrosol over your face.

✦ ✦ ✦ ✦

APOTHECARY TIP

Do not discard the herbal water after your treatment. You can add the infusion to your evening bath for a rejuvenating soak.

✦ ✦ ✦ ✦

Choosing Herbs for Your Skin Type:

For oily skin that is prone to acne, prepare a calendula, sage, or yarrow infusion.
For dry skin, prepare a chamomile, parsley, or fresh mint infusion.

Here's how to prepare your herbal infusion:
Add 2 tablespoons of herbs to a cup of boiling water. Let steep for 15 minutes.
Strain and let cool.

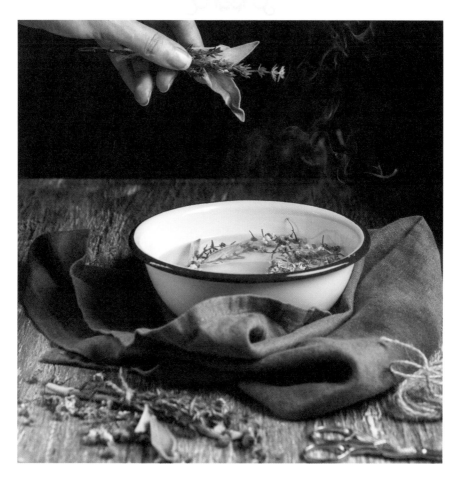

POMEGRANATE AND ROSE HIP WHIPPED MOISTURIZER

Natural moisturizers can slow down the evaporation of your skin's moisture while protect tiny fissures in your skin from damaging environments. Loaded with antioxidants and fatty acids from both the pomegranate and the rose hips, plus the antimicrobial properties of coconut oil, this powerful free radical–fighting moisturizer is your best solution for age-defying skin.

MAKES 5 OUNCES

½ cup coconut oil
1 tablespoon pomegranate powder
1 tablespoon rose hip oil

Heat the coconut oil in a double boiler or a heat-safe bowl perched over a saucepan of simmering water and stir in the pomegranate powder. Allow to infuse for 20 minutes. Add the rose hip oil and remove from the heat.

Let the oil cool until it is almost solid, then, using a handheld electric mixer or a fork, whip the oil until a beautiful pink cream is formed. Transfer to a lidded glass jar.

To use: Apply with your fingertips and massage the cream into your skin as needed.

Store in its sealed glass jar in the refrigerator. For maximum freshness and potency, please use within 6 months.

APOTHECARY TIP

Pomegranate powder is dried and ground pomegranate arils. Because it is freeze-dried, it is raw, preserving nutrients and enzymes. You can find pomegranate powder in natural food stores as well as online.

✦ ✦ ✦ ✦

ROSE OIL ELIXIR

Rose oil is another versatile and extremely potent antibacterial oil infusion. Its anti-inflammatory and tissue-regenerating agents make it the perfect luxurious skin-replenishing elixir.

MAKES 4 OUNCES

6 tablespoons rose-infused almond oil
2 tablespoons vitamin E oil, or the contents of 5 capsules
5 to 10 drops rose essential oil (optional)

Stir together the oils in a lidded glass jar and allow to synergize in a dark location for 24 hours.

To use: Apply the elixir to your face, after cleansing, while your skin is still damp. Massage into your skin, beginning with your décolletage, throat, then your face, using circular, upward, and outward strokes.

Store in its sealed glass jar in a cool, dark place. For maximum freshness and potency, please use within 6 months.

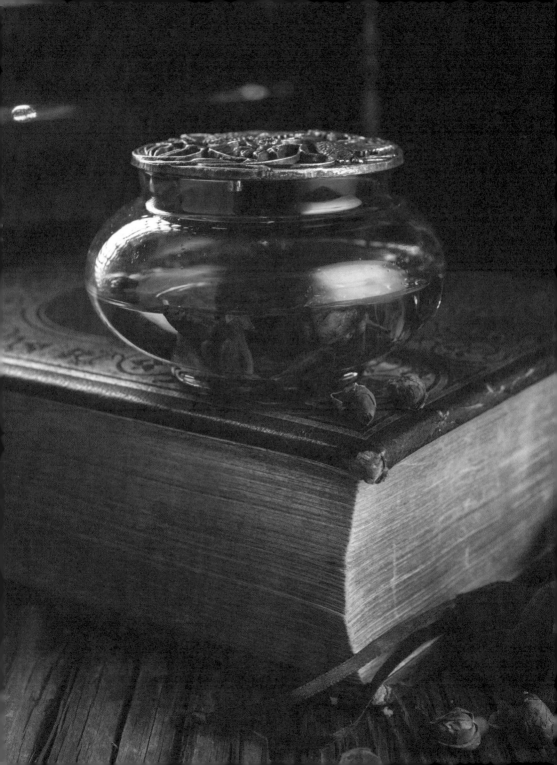

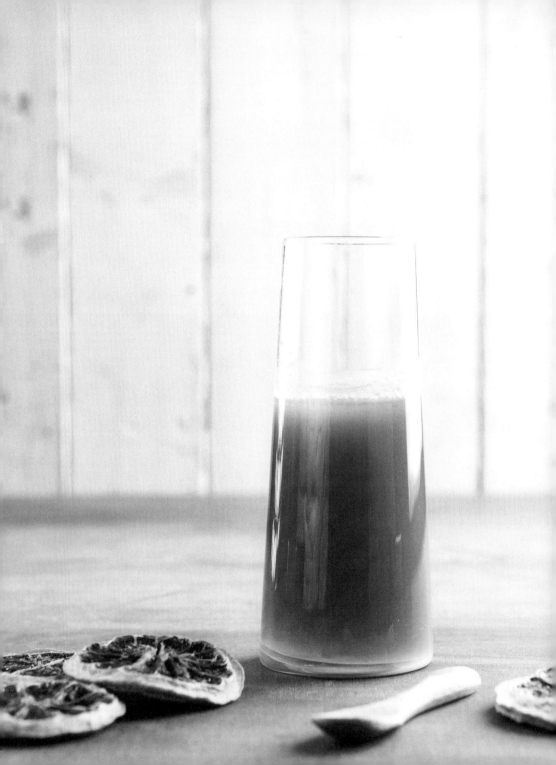

VITAMIN C LOVE SERUM

Help boost your complexion and fight the signs of stress by increasing your skin's circulation with this powerful serum. Using the vitamin C–rich lemon juice and the Amazonian wonder fruit camu-camu at its base, as well as the addition of aloe vera and glycerin, makes this a powerful solution for radiant and refreshed skin.

MAKES 2½ OUNCES

1 teaspoon warm distilled water
1 teaspoon fresh lemon juice
1 teaspoon camu-camu powder
2 tablespoons aloe vera gel
1 tablespoon vegetable glycerin

Mix together the warm water and lemon juice in a small bowl and add the camu-camu powder, allowing the powder to dissolve completely. Then, using a funnel, pour the mixture into a small, lidded glass jar, adding the aloe vera gel and glycerin. Close the lid and shake to combine the ingredients.

To use: Smooth a small amount over your face, neck, and chest. Allow to absorb into your skin.

Store in its sealed glass jar in the refrigerator. For maximum freshness and potency, please use within 1 week.

FACIAL MASSAGE 101

About 30 muscles are linked together beneath the skin of the face and head. We use most of these muscles every day. Repetitive muscle expansions and contractions can deplete our skin and lead to an accumulation of toxins. Regular massage can increase blood circulation and improve both the firmness and resilience of our skin. Always approach your face with a gentle and mindful touch.

Follow this simple technique to give yourself regular facial massages:

Begin by applying facial oil to your hands. Rub the formula between your palms to heat the oil and to evenly distribute it over your hands and fingertips. If you're dealing with a specific skin issue you'd like to heal, set a healing intention before you begin. This can be a phrase spoken in first person, present tense, such as: I wash away all that does not serve me.

Press your oiled fingers between your brows and slide them toward your temples, repeating several times to cover the entire area.

Massage your upper eyelids by sliding your fingers outward from the bridge of your nose. For your lower eyelids, slide your fingers outward in an arc as if ironing out the fine lines at the corners of your eyes. Finish by sliding your fingers down toward the outer sides of your cheeks.

Continue by sliding your fingers downward along the bridge of your nose, then move your fingers carefully up and down along the outside of your nostrils.

Around your mouth, massage above and below your lips in turn, sliding your fingers outward from the center.

On your cheeks, move your fingers in a spiral direction from your jawline up to your temples.

Stroke the nape of your neck downward toward your chest.

To end, gently place your hands over your face and take a few deep, relaxing breaths. With each exhalation, feel your body release whatever you're holding on to that doesn't serve you.

Then, slide your hands outward toward the bottoms of your ears. Gently pull your earlobes. Release and relax.

ACAI BERRY FACIAL MASK

This fresh, vibrant facial mask is a delight for your skin. I like to think of it as a smoothie for your face. The gentle exfoliating action of the textured banana and nourishing avocado oil assists in removing debris trapped in pores, while the double nourishing benefits of both the blackberry and acai berry, rich in polyphenols, work to tighten skin and minimize pores. Adding just a touch of lemon juice can also help exfoliate and improve vitamin C absorption.

MAKES 1 TREATMENT

½ banana
1 teaspoon acai powder
5 whole fresh blackberries
1 teaspoon avocado oil

Place the banana, acai powder, and berries in a blender and blend, then slowly add the oil and blend again.

To use: Massage onto your face, neck, and chest and leave on for 15 minutes, then rinse with warm water.

For maximum freshness and potency, please use immediately.

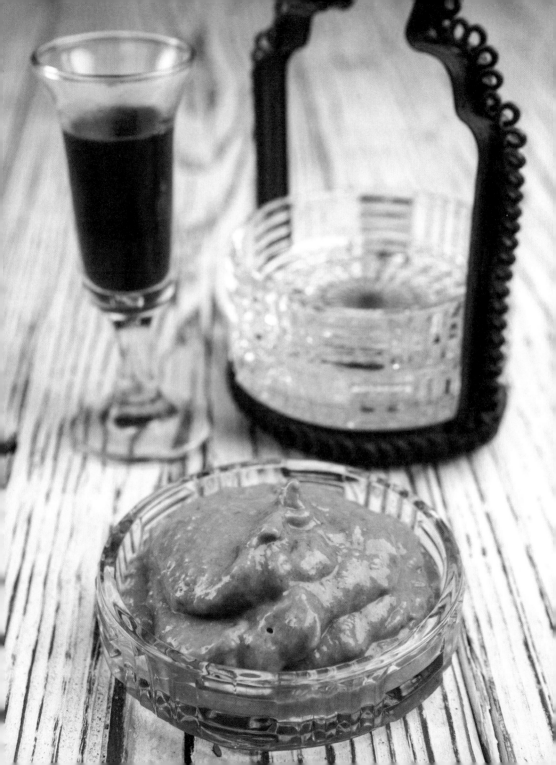

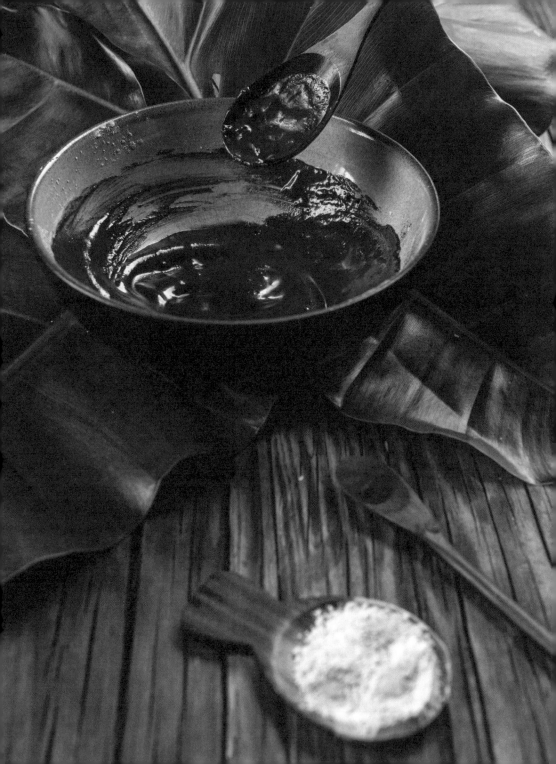

SEA SIREN MASK

Three powerful ingredients work in harmony in this luxurious sea mask. The French green clay coaxes out deep toxins, the mineral-rich spirulina clears out blemishes and fights free radicals, while the moisturizing coconut oil nourishes and replenishes skin for a soothing and softening seaside treat worthy of a siren.

MAKES ABOUT 6 MASKS

2 ounces French green clay
1 tablespoon spirulina powder

PER APPLICATION
2 tablespoons distilled water
1 teaspoon coconut oil

Mix together the clay and spirulina powder in a lidded glass jar.

To use: Mix 2 teaspoons of the clay mixture with the water and coconut oil in a small bowl to create a muddy paste. Apply the mask all over your face, neck, and chest, avoiding the skin around your eyes. Leave on for 15 minutes, then rinse with warm water.

Store the dry mixture in its sealed glass jar in a cool, dark place. For maximum freshness and potency, please use within 1 year.

✦ ✦ ✦ ✦

APOTHECARY TIP

Once you apply the mask to the skin, spritz your face with a hydrating toner, such as the Apple and Green Tea Face Toner (page 59) or the Grapefruit Vanilla Face Mist (page 60), to ensure that it stays active and your skin reaps the most benefits.

✦ ✦ ✦ ✦

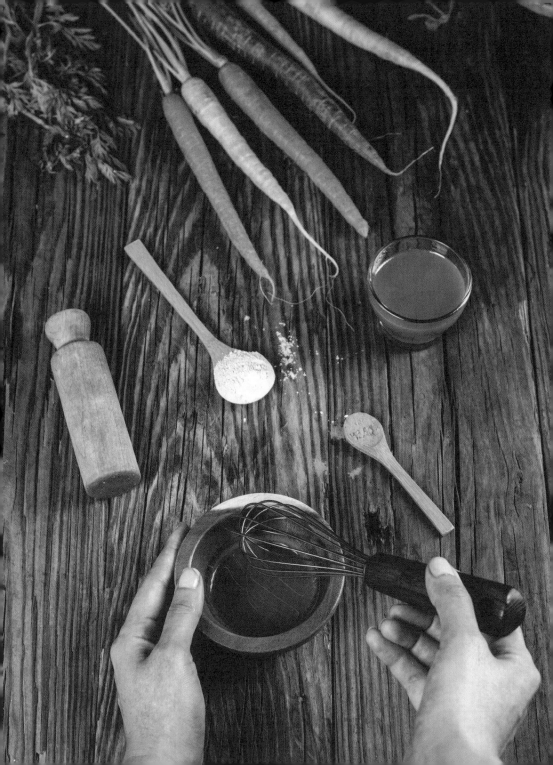

BEAUTY CARROT MASK

Carrots are rich in vitamin A, an important beauty vitamin instrumental in maintaining healthy skin and hair. Fresh carrot juice and turmeric also have strong antiseptic properties that can help clear up blemished skin. Use this simple, nourishing mask anytime you need to brighten, exfoliate, and calm inflamed skin.

MAKES 1 TO 2 APPLICATIONS

¼ cup carrot juice
1 teaspoon ground turmeric
¼ cup kaolin clay

Mix together all the ingredients in a small bowl, remembering to use wooden or ceramic tools and bowls when working with clay.

To use: Spread the mixture over clean skin and let sit for 15 to 20 minutes. Rinse with warm water.

For maximum freshness and potency, please use immediately.

PAPAYA FACE SCRUB

Papayas are a very rich source of antioxidants, essential for skin health. Rich in alpha hydroxy acids, they offer excellent antiaging properties, while the fruit enzymes assist in new cell regeneration. Papaya seeds, often discarded, also have wonderful antiseptic properties, making them an excellent natural scrub. The next time you are enjoying this tropical fruit, remember to keep the seeds to make this incredibly simple and delightful age-fighting and skin-brightening treatment.

MAKES 1 TREATMENT

2 tablespoons papaya seeds
1 tablespoon papaya fruit
1 teaspoon olive oil

Place all the ingredients in a high-speed blender and blend, to grind the seeds and make a puree.

To use: Massage gently onto skin to exfoliate. Leave on for 15 minutes, then rinse with warm water.

For maximum freshness and potency, please use immediately.

✦ ✦ ✦ ✦

BEAUTY NOTE

Papaya is known for promoting clear, healthy skin both from the inside and out. The seeds are edible and are particularly potent. Spicy papaya seeds can be dried, crushed, and used in place of black pepper to season foods. Add them to your diet slowly so as not to overwhelm your digestive system.

✦ ✦ ✦ ✦

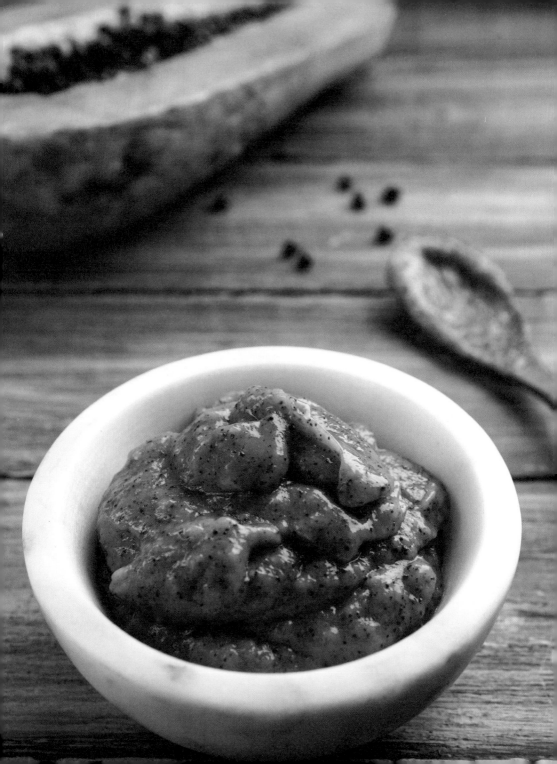

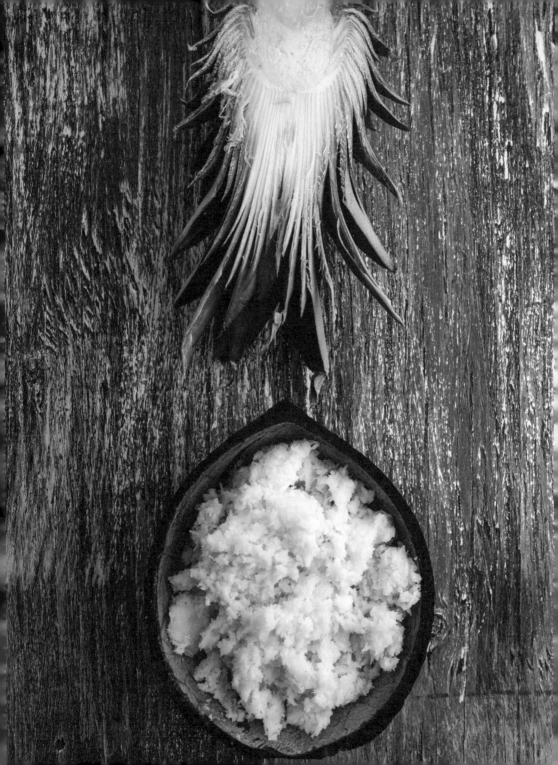

PIÑA COLADA FACE POLISH

This enchanting tropical concoction, reminiscent of your favorite getaway cocktail, is full of healthy fat and vitamins, to nourish and gently exfoliate your parched skin. Use whenever you need a dose of island life.

MAKES I TO 2 APPLICATIONS

¼ cup pineapple
1½ teaspoons pure coconut milk
1½ tablespoons coconut oil
¼ cup dried shredded coconut

Combine the pineapple, coconut milk, and coconut oil in a high-speed blender and blend until smooth. Mix in the shredded coconut for texture and transfer to a lidded glass jar.

To use: Massage gently onto your skin to exfoliate. Leave on for 15 minutes, preferably while sipping on an alcoholic version. Rinse with warm water.

Store in its sealed glass jar in the refrigerator. For maximum freshness and potency, please use within 1 week.

STRAWBERRIES AND CREAM FACE POLISH

The next best thing to eating strawberries? Why, it's putting them on your face, of course! Not only are strawberries rich in vitamin C, they are also great sources of salicylic acid, protecting the skin from environmental stressors. In conjunction with the antioxidant powerhouse that are goji berries, this beautiful face polish will help you maintain healthy, dewy, youthful skin.

MAKES 1 TREATMENT

1 tablespoon coconut cream (see instructions below)
¼ cup hulled strawberries
1 tablespoon goji berries

Without shaking it, open a can of organic coconut milk and scoop out only the rich cream accumulated on top. Place the coconut cream in a blender, add the strawberries and goji berries, and blend until you create a scrublike mixture.

To use: Massage gently onto your skin to exfoliate. Leave on for 15 minutes, then rinse with warm water.

For maximum freshness and potency, please use immediately.

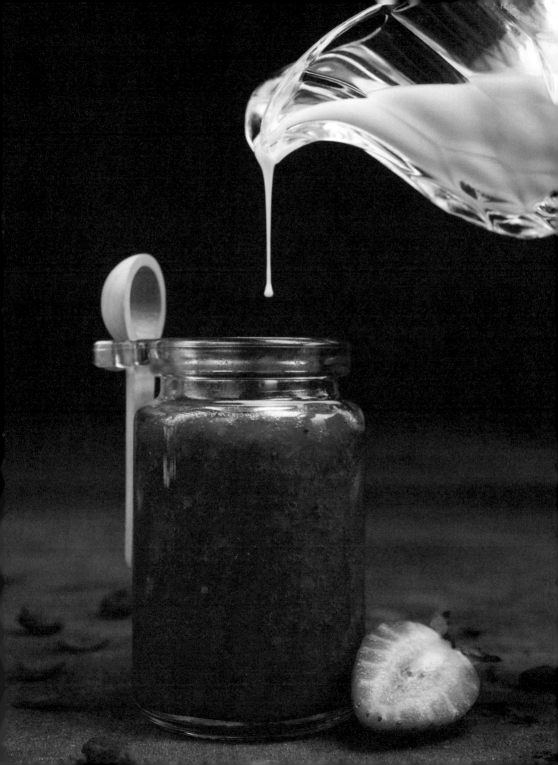

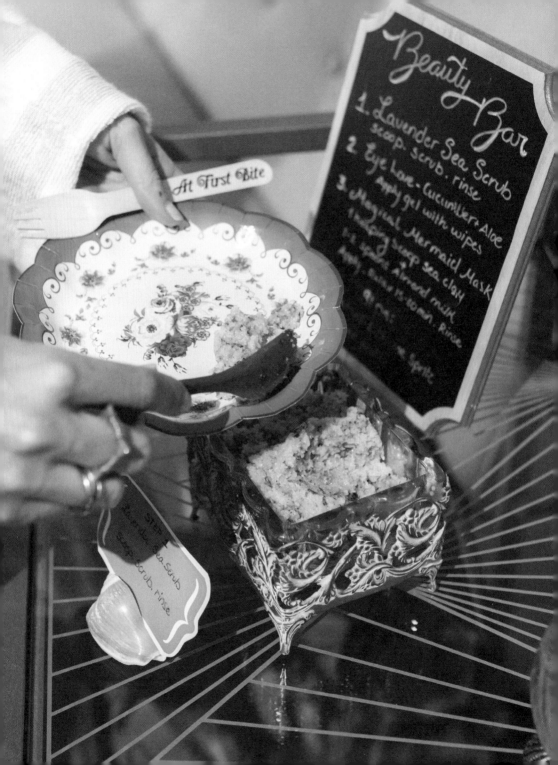

APPLE AND GREEN TEA FACE TONER

Apple cider vinegar is a rock star natural beauty ingredient. It delivers beneficial vitamins, minerals, and amino acids deep into the skin. Green tea, with high levels of polyphenols and catechins, is a superstar in its own right, drawing out impurities and improving the skin's elasticity. Go ahead, spritz on the superpower protection.

MAKES 10 OUNCES

2 teaspoons green tea leaves, or 2 tea bags
1 cup hot water
¼ cup raw apple cider vinegar
10 drops bergamot, citrus, or rose essential oil (optional)

Steep the green tea in the hot water for 10 minutes. Remove and discard the tea leaves or bags and allow the infusion to cool to room temperature. Add the vinegar and essential oils and transfer to a lidded glass jar.

To use: Apply the toner with a cotton ball or transfer the mixture to a spray bottle and spritz as needed.

Store in its sealed glass jar or spray bottle in the refrigerator. For maximum freshness and potency, please use within 3 months.

GRAPEFRUIT VANILLA FACE MIST

Nothing beats a refreshing mist on a hot day. Spritz on the cooling aloe and the stimulating citrus blend for a hydrating dose of topical refreshment. Bonus: The antibacterial and anti-inflammatory properties of aloe vera juice can help with minor cuts and burns.

MAKES 10 OUNCES

¾ cup distilled water
¼ cup aloe vera juice
1 teaspoon pure vanilla extract
Juice of ½ grapefruit

Mix all the ingredients together in a small bowl and, using a funnel, transfer the liquid to a spray bottle.

To use: Spritz on your face after cleansing and whenever you need a quick pick-me-up during the day.

Store in its spray bottle in the refrigerator. For maximum freshness and potency, please use within 3 months.

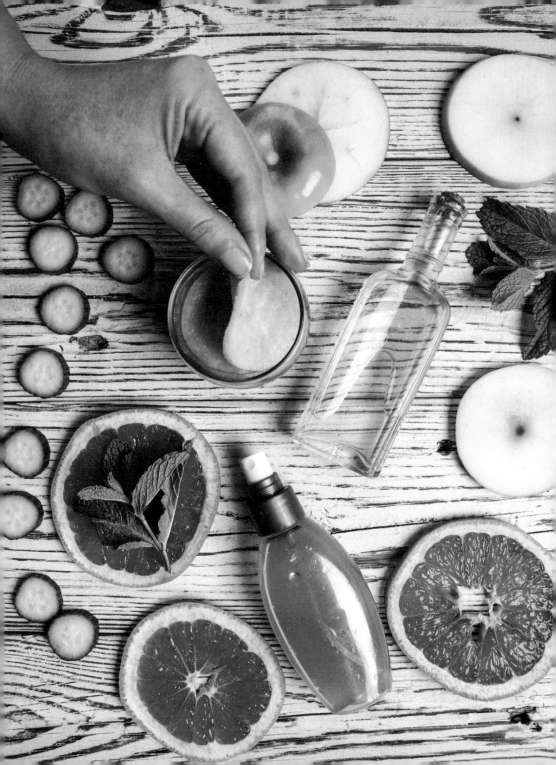

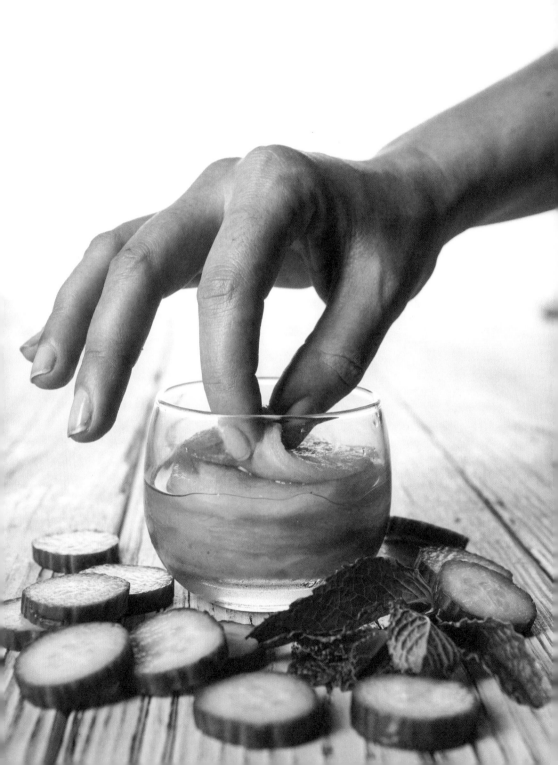

CUCUMBER MINT ALOE FACE WIPES

Full of antioxidants, these cooling and refreshing face wipes make it easy to sweep away grime on the go, leaving skin feeling refreshed and revived.

MAKES 10 OUNCES

½ cup witch hazel
½ cup cucumber juice
⅓ cup aloe vera gel
2 drops peppermint essential oil

Stack 30 cotton face wipes in a 10-ounce lidded, wide-mouth glass jar. (Alternatively, you can choose to keep the liquid mixture free of pads and use a cotton ball to apply as needed.)

Combine all the ingredients in a small bowl, then slowly pour the mixture over the pads, until they are fully saturated. Close the lid of the jar and allow the pads to soak up the mixture for at least an hour.

To use: Pick up a wipe and smooth over your face for a clean sweep.

Store in its sealed glass jar in the refrigerator. For maximum freshness and potency, please use within 3 months.

Don't Neglect Your Neck

*Your skin care routine shouldn't stop at your chin.
It should extend all the way down to your décolletage,
that sexy cleavage area always revealed by a low
neckline. All the face cleansers, moisturizers, scrubs,
and masks in this book are gentle enough to be used on
both your neck and décolletage.*

*To best apply your face products on the sensitive skin
of the neck, while looking upward to keep the skin taut,
apply the product to the front and sides of your neck
and massage lightly in circular motions for 1 minute.
(Looking upward while massaging your neck will tighten
the skin and make application easier.) When exfoliating,
take care not to press too hard, as the skin on your neck
is more sensitive than the skin on your face.*

NECK-SMOOTHING COMPRESS

¼ cup dried chamomile flowers
1 cup almond milk
2 tablespoons avocado oil

Combine the chamomile flowers and almond milk in a small saucepan and bring to a boil. Remove from the heat, allow to cool slightly, and strain the infusion.

To use: Lather avacado oil generously to cover the entire neck. Dip a small towel or thick cloth into the infusion and apply the warm mixture around your neck. Superimpose plastic wrap and a dry towel over the compress and keep on for 20 minutes.

For maximum freshness and potency, please use immediately.

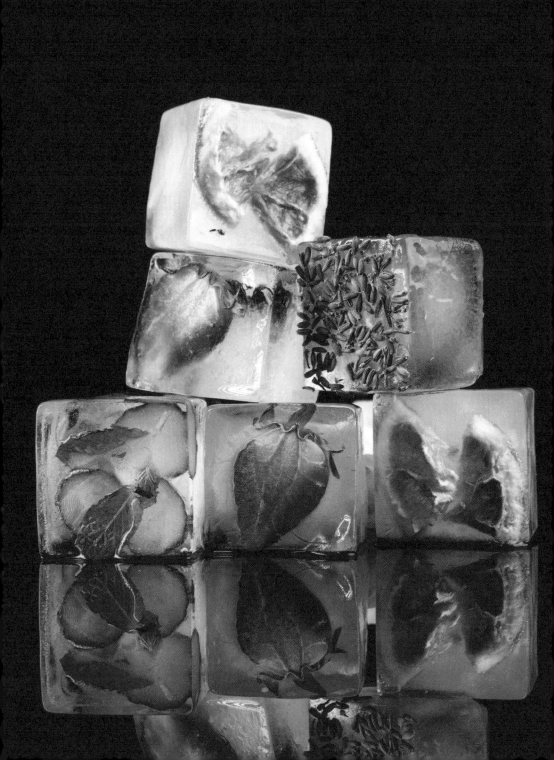

ICE QUEEN BEAUTY THERAPY

Who would have thought that the little icy jewel we use to cool our drinks could do such wonders for our skin?! From relieving sunburn and reducing puffy eyes to giving us an instant face lift, ice has played an important role in beauty rituals for centuries.

Queen Catherine II of Russia was well known for using ice on her face, neck, and décolletage every morning, to preserve her beauty and refresh her complexion.

You, too, can incorporate a simple, icy beauty treatment into your morning routine, to revitalize and restore natural dewiness to your skin.

The process is simple and the combinations are simply endless. Aloe vera and cucumber will soothe sunburned skin. The caffeine and antioxidants in green tea will work wonders on puffy, tired eyes. Lemon will brighten and revive the complexion; lavender and rose water will calm inflamed skin.

To prepare, simply brew a cup of strong tea or herbs to create an infusion, add pureed fruits or veggies, and add aloe, coconut water, and additional nutritious ingredients of your choice. Allow to cool and pour into ice cube trays.

To use, gently and quickly wipe your face, neck, and décolletage with a Beauty Queen ice cube, using the facial massage techniques on pages 44–46. Please note that when using ice cubes on the delicate skin on your face, you must be quite gentle, so as to protect the blood vessels and capillaries under the skin. Alternatively, wrap the ice cube in a light, soft cloth.

◆ ◆ ◆ ◆

BEAUTY NOTE

To get even more benefits from your ice cube treatment, add ½ teaspoon of your preferred carrier oil to your infusion before freezing it. Then, wipe your face and neck with these ice cubes before your makeup goes on. The addition of oil will soften and nourish your skin, preparing it for a smooth and flawless makeup application.

◆ ◆ ◆ ◆

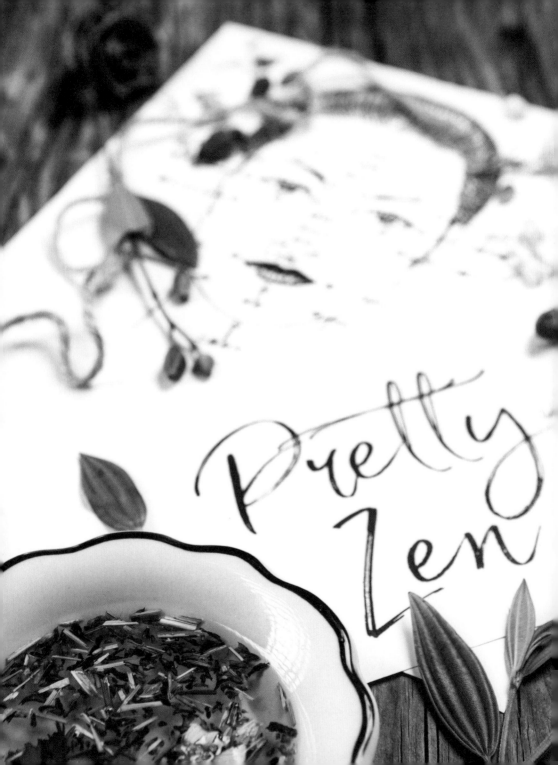

NOURISHING EYE BALM

Eyes are one of the most important organs in the body and one of the parts of the face we notice first. Take good care of them with this and the following loving recipes.

This nourishing balm, rich in antioxidants from the cranberries comingled with the healing moisture of vitamin E, is a loving way to give the sensitive skin around the eyes that fresh, lifted feeling it's been missing.

MAKES 1½ OUNCES

1 ounce shea butter
1 tablespoon cranberry seed oil
1 teaspoon vitamin E oil
5 drops rose essential oil (optional)

Melt the shea butter in a double boiler or a heat-safe bowl perched over a saucepan of simmering water, taking care not to overheat. Gently whisk in the cranberry oil. Remove from the heat and add the vitamin E and essential oils, if using.

Transfer the mixture to a lidded glass jar. Allow to cool before sealing the lid.

To use: Apply in the evening by carefully dabbing the balm around your eyes.

Store in its sealed glass jar in the refrigerator. For maximum freshness and potency, please use within 3 months.

COOLING EYE GEL

The delicate skin around the eyes is the thinnest on the whole body and is especially vulnerable to changes in appearance. This light, cooling treatment, made with soothing aloe vera gel and nourishing vitamin E oil, moisturizes the skin and repairs damaged cells in the gentlest way.

MAKES I TREATMENT

1 teaspoon aloe vera gel
1 teaspoon vitamin E oil
2 cucumber slices, large enough to cover the area of your eyes

Stir together the aloe vera gel and vitamin E oil in a small bowl.

To use: Dab gently on the skin around your eyes. Find a comfortable spot to recline and place the cucumber slices over your closed eyelids. Relax for 15 minutes before removing the cucumber and rinsing with water.

For maximum freshness and potency, please use immediately.

LASH SERUM

An eyelash grows for about six months before falling out. Treat your lashes with the following serum to keep them growing healthy, shiny, and conditioned.

MAKES 2 OUNCES

2 tablespoons castor oil
2 tablespoons aloe vera gel
1 teaspoon vitamin E oil

Combine all three ingredients in a small lidded glass jar.

To use: Shake the jar vigorously and apply the serum to your lashes every evening before bed.

Store in its sealed glass jar in the refrigerator. For maximum freshness and potency, please use within 3 months.

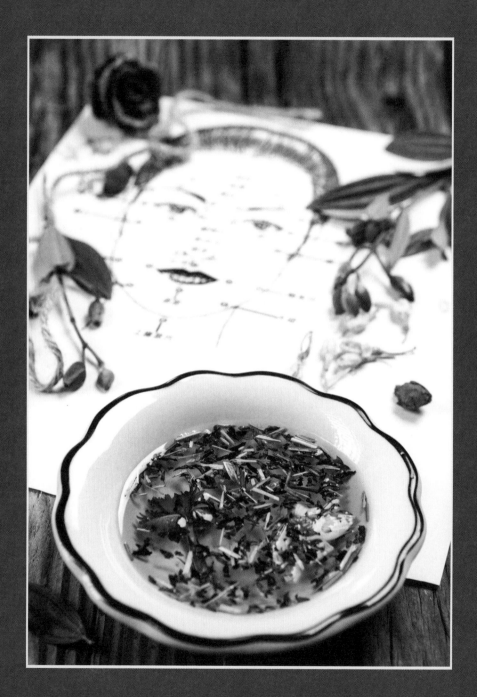

NATURAL MAKEUP

Finding makeup that's both effective and made without toxic chemicals can be difficult these days. Even the ever popular "natural" label, along with labels touting products as "clean," "pure," "green," and "eco-friendly," are not federally defined or regulated. It's up to you, as the consumer, to do your own diligent homework. In the meantime, here's a few staples you'll love making yourself.

Lime in the Coconut Lip Scrub

Moisture-Rich Lip Treatment

Chocolate Lip Butter

Lip and Cheek Stain

Custom Blush

Custom Sun-Kissed Bronzer

Eye-Friendly Mascara

Nontoxic Eyeliner

Eye Makeup Remover

THE DIRTY LIST

There is a great deal of freedom for the beauty industry in the formulation of cosmetics, making many of the ingredients in our makeup products decisively not so pretty. You can avoid most harsh chemicals, however, by making your own whenever possible. Here's a list of ingredients you should definitely stay clear of:

FORMALDEHYDE: Found in nail polish, hair and body cleansers, and eye shadows, formaldehyde-releasing preservatives (FRPs) are used to help prevent bacteria growth and has been deemed a human carcinogen by the International Agency Research on Carcinogens.

FRAGRANCE: Fragrance mixes in perfumes, colognes, and cleansers have been associated with allergies, dermatitis, respiratory distress, and can affect the reproductive system.

PARABENS: Parabens are widely used preservatives that possess estrogen-mimicking properties associated with increased risk of breast cancer and prostate cancer development.

PHTHALATES: Dibutyl phthalate in nail polish, diethyl phthalate in perfume, and dimethyl phthalate in hair spray are known endocrine disruptors linked to cancer and reproductive birth defects. As with fragrances, they do not have to be disclosed on product labels.

PROPYLENE GLYCOL: Propylene glycol is an organic alcohol commonly used as a skin-conditioning agent. It's classified as a skin irritant and penetrator. It has been associated with causing dermatitis as well as hives in humans— these sensitization effects can be manifested at propylene glycol concentrations as low as 2 percent. It can be found in moisturizers, sunscreens, makeup products, conditioners, shampoos, and hair sprays.

SODIUM LAURYL SULFATE (SLS): This surfactant can be found in more than 90 percent of personal care and cleaning products as a foaming agent. SLSs are known to be skin, lung, and eye irritants. A major concern about SLS is its potential to interact and combine with other chemicals to form nitrosamines, which are carcinogenic. These combinations can lead to a host of other issues, such as kidney and respiratory damage. They can be found in shampoos, body washes, cleansers, mascaras, and acne treatments.

SUNSCREEN CHEMICALS: These chemicals absorb ultraviolet light. They are also endocrine disruptors and are believed to be easily absorbed into the body. They may also cause cellular damage and cancer in the body. Common names are benzophenone, PABA, avobenzone, homosalate, and methoxycinnmate. They can be found in sunscreen products and in some facial foundations.

SYNTHETIC COLORS: "FD&C" or "D&C" represent artificial colors: F for "food" and D&C for "drug and cosmetics." These letters precede a color and number (e.g., D&C Red 27 or FD&C Blue 1). These synthetic colors are derived from petroleum or coal tar sources. They are considered human carcinogens by the European Classification and Labeling system and the European Union has banned them, but they are still quite prevalent in the United States.

TOLUENE: A petrochemical derived from petroleum or coal tar sources. You may see it listed on labels as benzene, toluol, phenylmethane, or methylbenzene. Toluene is a potent solvent able to dissolve paint. It can affect your respiratory system, cause nausea, and irritate your skin. Toluene has also been linked to immune system toxicity. It can be found in nail polish, nail treatments, and hair coloring/bleaching products.

TRICLOSAN: Triclosan is a widely used antimicrobial chemical that's a known endocrine disruptor, especially of thyroid and reproductive hormones, and a skin irritant. Studies raise concerns that triclosan contributes to making bacteria antibiotic-resistant. Triclosan can be found in toothpastes, antibacterial soaps, and deodorants.

For a complete list of substances to avoid, visit the Environmental Working Group (EWG) Skin Deep Database.

LIME IN THE COCONUT LIP SCRUB

The skin on the lips is like no other on the body: It's thinner—allowing the blood vessels to be visible and giving color to our puckers, and has no oil or sweat glands to protect it from the elements. This recipe and the ones that follow are carefully formulated to give your pretty mouth the best care.

This scrumptious lip scrub combines gentle exfoliation with much needed moisture to keep lips softer longer, even in the dead of winter; while the smell and the taste will most certainly transport you to a warm island far, far away.

MAKES ½ OUNCE

1 teaspoon coconut sugar
1 teaspoon fresh lime juice
1 teaspoon coconut oil

Combine all the ingredients in a small bowl and stir to form a smooth paste. Transfer to a lidded glass jar.

To use: Apply the mixture to your lips and massage gently to exfoliate. Rinse with warm water.

Store in its sealed glass jar in the refrigerator. For maximum freshness and potency, please use within 1 week.

MOISTURE-RICH LIP TREATMENT

Most commercial lip balms dry out the lips, which in turn makes us apply even more, turning us all into some sort of lip balm addict. For real relief from a dry, chapped pucker, try this tried-and-true overnight cure.

MAKES ½ OUNCE

1 teaspoon castor oil
1 teaspoon pure maple syrup
1 teaspoon fresh lemon juice

Stir together all the ingredients in a small bowl and transfer to a lidded glass jar.

To use: Spread the mixture on your lips and leave overnight.

Store in its sealed glass jar in the refrigerator. For maximum freshness and potency, please use within 1 week.

CHOCOLATE LIP BUTTER

This creamy and heavenly scented lip balm is so good, good luck trying not to eat it. Vitamin E and coconut oil deliver intensive healing, while cocoa butter and vegetable wax protect and seal in moisture.

MAKES 2 OUNCES

1 tablespoon vegetable wax
1 tablespoon cocoa butter
1 tablespoon coconut oil
1 teaspoon vitamin E oil
½ teaspoon pure vanilla extract
1 teaspoon cacao powder

Melt the wax and cocoa butter in a double boiler or a heat-safe bowl perched over a saucepan of simmering water. Add the coconut oil. Once all the ingredients have melted, remove from the heat. Add the vitamin E, vanilla, and cacao powder and mix thoroughly.

Carefully transfer the mixture to a lidded tin or glass jar. Leave the lid off until the balm has cooled completely.

To use: Apply with your fingertips whenever your lips need a little extra moisture.

Store in its sealed container in a cool, dry place. For maximum freshness and potency, please use within 6 months.

✦ ✦ ✦ ✦

BEAUTY NOTE

To add a pop of color to your lip butter and the prettiest crimson shade to lips, add ⅛ teaspoon of beet or hibiscus powder.

✦ ✦ ✦ ✦

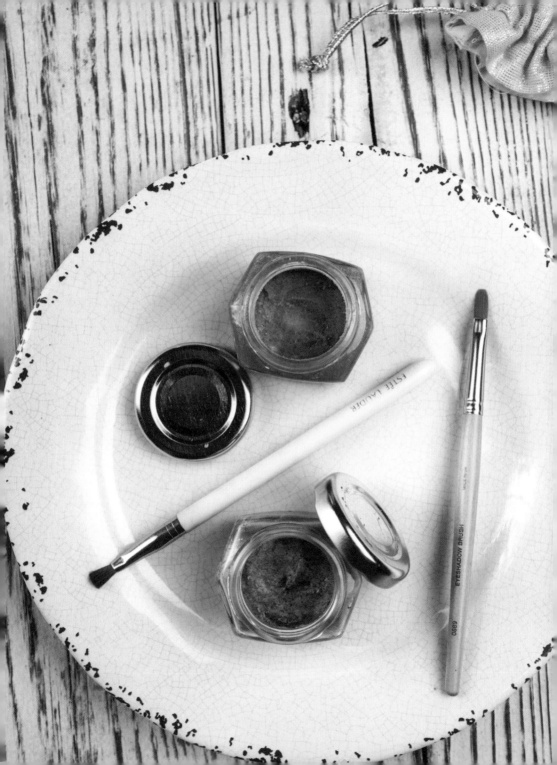

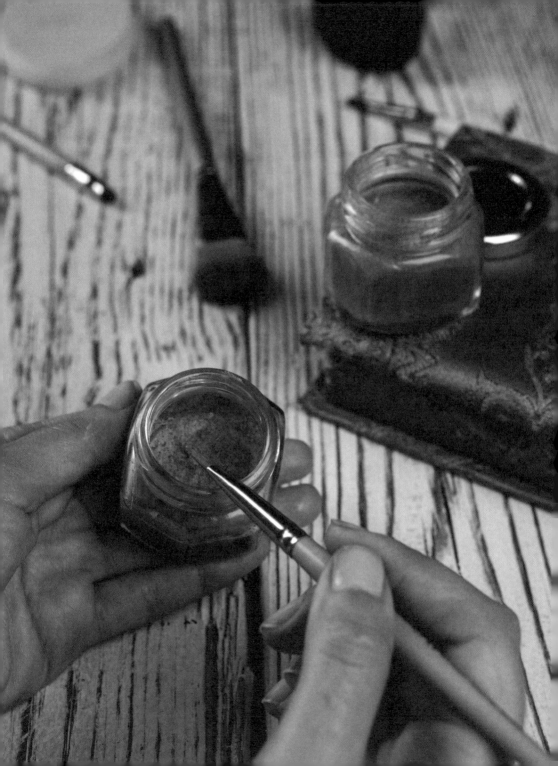

LIP AND CHEEK STAIN

This easy, three-ingredient lip and cheek stain makes the prettiest color for your face. Rub some on whenever you need a pop of color.

MAKES 2 OUNCES

2 tablespoons coconut oil
2 tablespoons beet powder
2 teaspoons shea butter

Melt the coconut oil in a double boiler or a heat-safe bowl perched over a saucepan of simmering water, then add the beet powder. Allow to infuse for 15 minutes, making sure not burn the mixture. Stir in the shea butter and mix until fully melted. Remove from the heat and allow the mixture to cool.

Once fully solidified, gently beat the mixture with a whisk until it is light and creamy. Transfer to a lidded glass jar or tin.

To use: Keep in your purse and apply on the go whenever you need a touch of color.

For maximum freshness and potency, please use within 6 months.

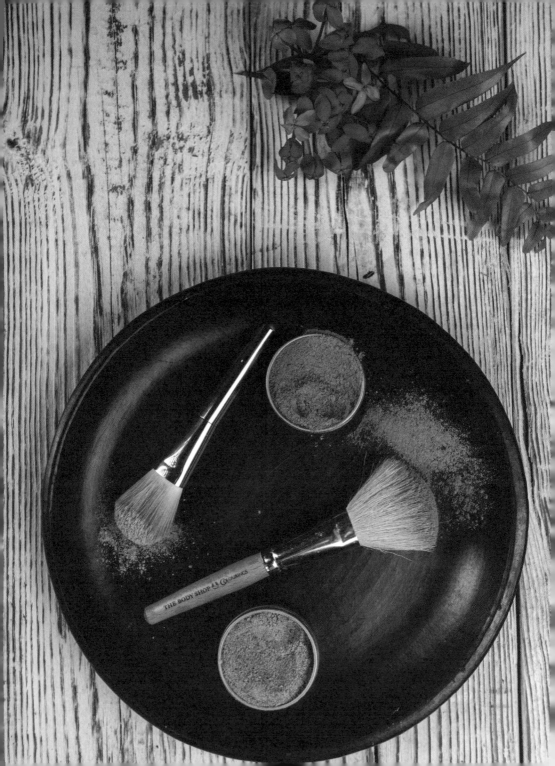

CUSTOM BLUSH

Your rosy cheeks await. Find your perfect shade and put a little color on your cheeks with this all-natural recipe you can feel good about.

MAKES ABOUT 1 TEASPOON

1 teaspoon tapioca or arrowroot flour
Beet powder
Cacao powder

Begin by mixing flour with 1 teaspoon of beet powder in a small bowl. Test this shade on your skin and begin adjusting it to your skin tone by adding more beet powder as needed. Experiment with cacao powder to create a darker hue. Once you are pleased with your custom shade, place the powder in a lidded glass container.

To use: Apply onto your cheekbones with your favorite blush brush.

Store in its sealed glass container in a cool, dry place. For maximum freshness and potency, please use within 6 months.

CUSTOM SUN-KISSED BRONZER

Your coveted summertime glow is here. This formula will put the sun back on your face in the safest way. Use it to sculpt and contour as well.

MAKES ABOUT I TEASPOON

1 teaspoon tapioca flour
Cacao powder
Ground cinnamon, nutmeg, turmeric, or beet powder

Begin by mixing the flour with the 1 teaspoon of cacao powder in a small bowl. Test this shade on your skin and begin adjusting it to your skin tone by adding more cacao powder as needed. Experiment with ground cinnamon or nutmeg to create a golden shimmer. You can also add ground turmeric or beet powder to find your perfect shade. Once you are pleased with your custom bronzer, place in a lidded glass container.

To use: Apply all over your face for a sun-kissed look or use to contour your face.

Store in its sealed glass container in a cool, dry place. For maximum freshness and potency, please use within 6 months.

EYE-FRIENDLY MASCARA

Beautiful eyelashes have long been associated with femininity. In fact, mascara dates back to ancient Egypt. Most formulas back then contained the same basic formula: pigmentation, oils, and waxes. The mascaras on the market today, however, contain methylparaben, aluminium powder, ceteareth-20, butylparaben, and benzyl alcohol, among others. This easy homemade formula will darken, separate, and condition your lovely lashes without the gunk.

MAKES ½ OUNCE

1 teaspoon activated charcoal
1 teaspoon bentonite clay
½ teaspoon plant-based glycerin
2 teaspoons aloe vera gel

Mix together all the ingredients in a small bowl until it reaches a smooth consistency. Transfer to a small lidded glass jar. (Alternatively, you can transfer the ingredients directly to a clean mascara tube and mix thoroughly with a clean mascara brush to get a smooth consistency.)

To use: Apply with a mascara brush whenever needed.

To remove: Use the eye makeup remover on page 87.

Store in its sealed container in a cool, dry place. For maximum freshness and potency, please use within 6 months.

✦ ✦ ✦ ✦

APOTHECARY TIP

If you prefer a more waterproof solution, replace the glycerin with vegetable wax. Follow the proper melting instructions for the wax before mixing with the other ingredients.

✦ ✦ ✦ ✦

NONTOXIC EYELINER

Some of us love our go-to liner. We use it every day, in the exact same way, and wouldn't dream of changing it up, but this natural liner might just be the tipping point to inspire you to break free from your toxic routine.

MAKES 1 OUNCE

2 teaspoons coconut oil
4 teaspoons aloe vera gel
½ teaspoon activated charcoal or the contents of 2 charcoal capsules
(for black), or ½ teaspoon cacao powder (for brown)

Thoroughly mix together all the ingredients in a small bowl and transfer to a small lidded tin or glass jar.

To use: Apply to your eyes, using a clean brush.

Store in its sealed container in a cool, dry place. For maximum freshness and potency, please use within 6 months.

EYE MAKEUP REMOVER

See that long list of ingredients on the back of your makeup remover? Some probably aren't as safe as you'd hope. This wonderfully mild recipe, on the other hand, will work to nourish your cherished peepers while removing even the toughest waterproof formulas.

MAKES 6 OUNCES

1 chamomile tea bag
¼ cup water
¼ cup wheat germ oil
¼ cup witch hazel

Combine the chamomile tea bag and the water in a small saucepan, bring to a boil, remove from the heat, and allow to steep for 10 minutes. Discard the tea bag and allow the infusion to cool. Add the wheat germ oil and witch hazel and transfer to a lidded glass jar.

To use: Shake well and pour a few drops of the solution onto a cotton ball. Wipe off your makeup gently without pulling at your lids.

Store in its sealed glass jar in the refrigerator. For maximum freshness and potency, please use within 3 months.

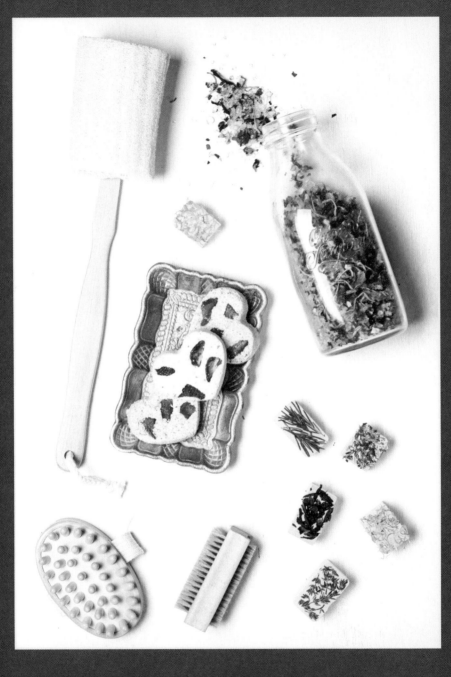

BODY CARE

Your body works hard for you on a daily basis. Pamper and indulge it with aromatic cleansers, invigorating bath salts, exfoliating scrubs, nourishing body butters, and luxurious body oils.

Personalized Botanical Soaps

Jasmine-Tangerine Body Wash

Tea Time Body Cleansing Powder

Luxurious Milky Bath

Cinnamon Ginger Sore Muscles Soak

Sleepy Time Herbal Tea Sachets

Dreamy Blue Bath Salts

Herbal Rose Bath Salts

Caressing Calendula Bath Salts

Rock Star Salts

Strawberry Love Bath Bombs

You're the Bomb Aromatherapy Shower Tablets

Chai Exfoliating Lotion Bars

Coffee Body Scrub

Luscious Mango Body Polish

Detoxifying Charcoal Body Scrub

Sea Mud Firming Body Wrap

Orange Blossom and Lemon Balm Body Lotion

Chocolate Soufflé Body Butter

Warming Vanilla Body Oil

Perfume Balm

Sensual Massage Oil

PERSONALIZED BOTANICAL SOAPS

These pretty jeweled soaps are a simple way to customize your bathing experience. If you've never made soap before, start here. Enjoy personalizing your soaps. They make wonderful gifts.

MAKES 16 OUNCES

Grapeseed oil or any neutral natural oil, for molds
16 ounces glycerin soap base
½ cup assorted dried botanicals
10 to 20 drops essential oils of your choice

Select your preferred soap molds and prepare them by greasing them with oil.

Grate the glycerin soap and place it in a double boiler or a heat-safe bowl perched over a pan of simmering water. Allow the soap to fully melt. Remove from the heat. Add the essential oils, if using, and stir to prevent bubbles from forming.

Arrange your chosen herbs and flowers in the bottom of your molds and pour the melted glycerin soap base over them.

Allow to cool and set for a few hours before removing the soap from the molds.

Keep in a closed container in a cool, dry place. For maximum freshness and potency, please use within 6 months.

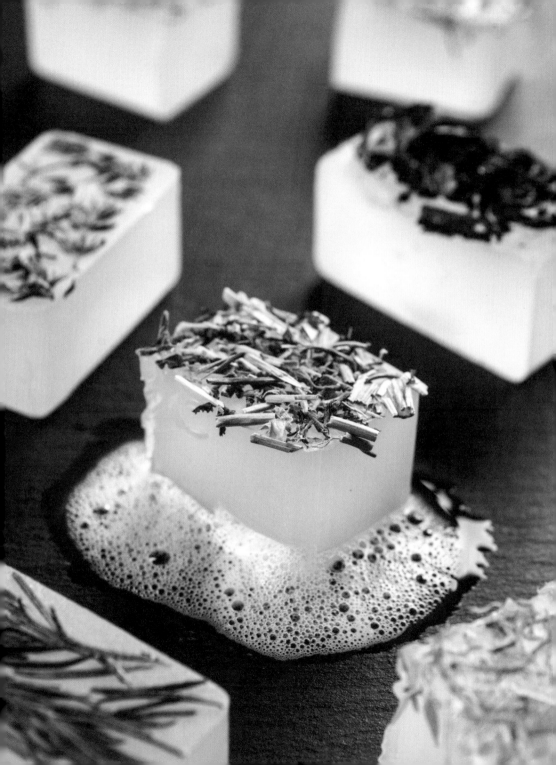

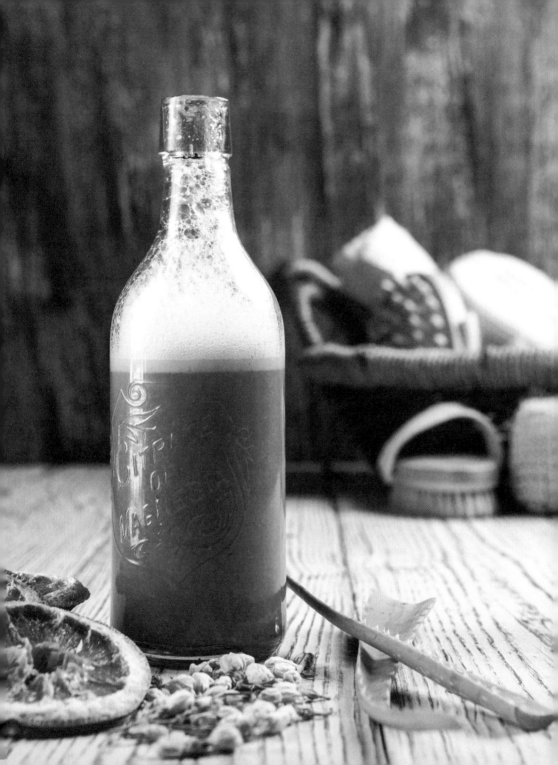

JASMINE-TANGERINE BODY WASH

This sudsy, sensual body wash feels great and smells even better. Lather on for an invigorating experience.

MAKES 10 OUNCES

1 tangerine
2 jasmine tea bags
½ cup distilled water
2 tablespoons coconut oil
½ cup Castile soap
2 tablespoons glycerin
15 drops jasmine essential oil

Juice the tangerine and keep the peel. Set the juice aside. Place the peel in a bowl along with the jasmine tea bags. Boil the distilled water and pour over the peel and tea bags. Allow to steep for 30 minutes, then strain the infusion. Allow the mixture to cool.

Melt the coconut oil in a double boiler or a heat-safe bowl perched over a saucepan of simmering water. Combine the Castile soap, glycerin, and melted coconut oil in a bowl. Add the tea mixture, jasmine essential oils, and the reserved tangerine juice. Using a funnel, transfer the mixture to a lidded glass bottle and swirl to mix the ingredients.

To use: Pour into your hands, lather onto your body, and rinse with warm water.

Store in its sealed bottle in the refrigerator. For maximum freshness and potency, please use within 3 months.

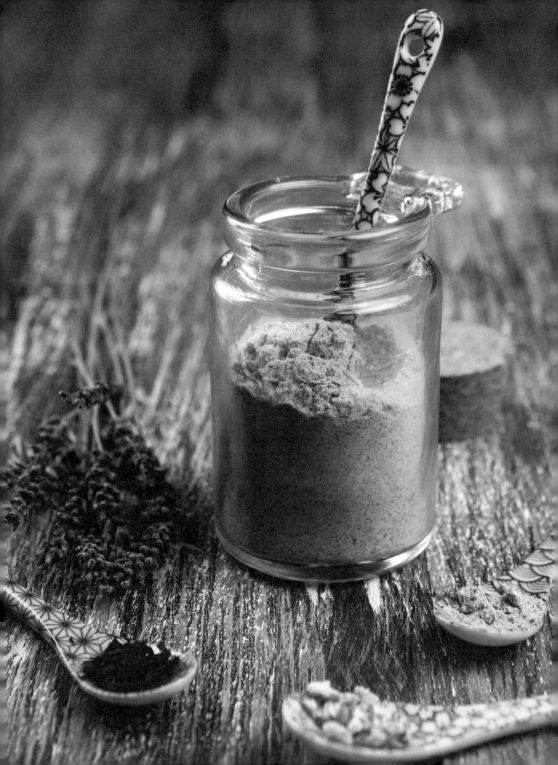

TEA TIME BODY CLEANSING POWDER

The haunting aromas of black tea, lavender, and orange zest intermingle with oatmeal to create a soothing and delightful cleansing experience.

MAKES 2 CUPS

½ cup rolled oats
¼ cup lavender buds
¼ cup orange zest
½ cup black tea leaves
½ cup white clay
Purified water

Place the oats, lavender buds, orange zest, and black tea in a spice or coffee grinder and grind to a fine powder. Mix with the clay and transfer to a lidded glass jar.

To use: Moisten your skin and massage the powder over your entire body, using circular motions, to soften dry skin cells. Rinse with warm water.

Store in its sealed glass jar in a cool, dark place. For maximum freshness and potency, please use within 6 months.

✦ ✦ ✦ ✦

APOTHECARY TIP

To use this enchanting tea cleanser as a mask, apply a thin layer all over your body and allow to dry for 20 minutes, then rinse with warm water.

✦ ✦ ✦ ✦

LUXURIOUS MILKY BATH

Cleopatra was known for taking long, luxurious, milky soaks to keep her skin soft and smooth. Pamper, soothe, and rejuvenate like a queen in these skin conditioning waters.

MAKES I BATH

1½ tablespoons dried lavender buds
1½ tablespoons dried rosemary
Peel of 1 orange
1 cup boiling water
1½ cups pure coconut milk

Combine the herbs and orange peel in a large pot and pour the boiling water over them. Allow to steep for a minimum of 2 hours or overnight.

Strain out the solids, keeping the infused liquid. Draw a bath and add the coconut milk and infused liquid to the tub.

Soak in the tub for a minimum of 20 minutes.

Shower and Bath Treatments

Whether you prefer a bath or shower, bathing is an opportunity to nurture yourself, reflect, and enjoy a much needed moment of pure, relaxing solitude. Beyond cleansing the body, it is a time and place to wash away the cares of the day. With the intention to unplug, use these recipes to experience the beauty of a bathing ritual at home.

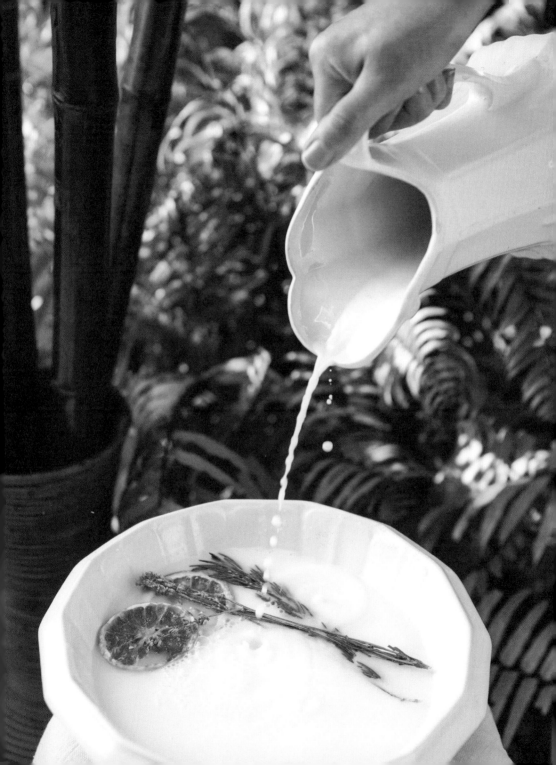

CINNAMON GINGER SORE MUSCLES SOAK

Ease your aches and pains with this toxin-fighting, muscle-soothing bath soak.

MAKES I BATH

1 cup raw apple cider vinegar
2 tablespoons sea salt
2 tablespoons baking soda
1 tablespoon ground cinnamon
1 tablespoon finely ground or grated fresh ginger
5 drops orange essential oil (optional)

Combine all the ingredients in a bowl and stir well. Add to your bath under running hot water, and soak for 20 minutes.

SLEEPY TIME HERBAL TEA SACHETS

Filling paper tea filters with skin-soothing ingredients, such as herbs, spices, salts, and essential oils, is a lovely way to treat yourself to a heavenly bath, without the need for much cleanup. These lovely aromatic bathing tea bags make a darling gift.

MAKES 8 TEA BAGS

1 cup Epsom salts
1 cup rolled oats
1 tablespoon dried chamomile flowers
1 tablespoon dried lavender buds
10 drops lavender essential oil
10 drops chamomile essential oil

Have 8 tea filter bags ready. Mix all the ingredients together in a medium bowl. Fill each tea bag with ¼ cup of the mixture.

To use: Add one tea bag to a warm bath. Soak in the tea bath for a minimum of 20 minutes to soothe sore muscles and detoxify.

Store the bags in a lidded glass jar or other container in a cool, dry place. For maximum freshness and potency, please use within 6 months.

ELEVATE YOUR BATHING EXPERIENCE

A comforting bath detoxifies, relaxes muscles, restores the body, and pampers the skin as you soak. And with a few extra steps, an otherwise average bath becomes a spa treatment tailored to the needs of your body, mind, and spirit.

+ Set the mood by dimming the lights and playing soft, meditative music.

+ Surround yourself with things of beauty that may help you relax, such as fresh flowers, energizing crystals, and candles.

+ Prepare your bath following any of the recipes on pages 96–99.

+ While your bath fills with warm water, exfoliate using a dry brush, to detoxify and soothe your skin while stimulating your blood flow.

+ Slowly slip into the bath, allowing your body to adjust to the temperature. Try to soak for at least 15 to 20 minutes.

+ Keep a glass of water and an aromatic mist, such as the Grapefruit Vanilla Face Mist (page 60) close by. A few mists onto your face and shoulders makes for a lovely midbath refresher.

+ Relax and let go of your thoughts and cares. Be present and enjoy the moment.

+ Exiting the bath, take a moment to ground yourself. Feel both feet rooted firmly on the floor. Take a few deep breaths and splash cool water on your face. Rehydrate with a glass of water.

+ Nourish your skin with body oil (see page 128). Slather it on and take time to connect with your body and nurture your skin. Pay extra attention to the places that need it most.

Showering can be the same relaxing ritual experience, using the You're the Bomb Aromatherapy Shower Tablets (pages 112–113). Shower tablets are the shower alternative to a relaxing, fragrant bath. Follow the same steps as above, using a shower tablet instead of taking a bath. Enjoy the aromatic essential oil blends as they disperse into the steam. Stop, relax, breathe, and connect with yourself. Stay in the moment and enjoy your ritual. Exit the shower the same way you would a bath. Reconnect and take a moment before easing yourself back into the day.

DREAMY BLUE BATH SALTS

Bath salts, in their purest form, contain many beneficial minerals, including magnesium, potassium, calcium, bromide, and, of course, sodium, that keep your skin mineralized, detoxified, and soothed.

MAKES 1½ CUPS

1 cup Dead Sea salt
½ cup dried lavender buds
1 tablespoon dried rosemary
1 teaspoon dried pea flowers
5 drops sage essential oil
5 drops lavender essential oil

Mix the ingredients thoroughly in a medium bowl. Add 1½ cups of bath salts to a standard-sized tub while the water is running, to help it dissolve. Fill tub ¾ full of warm water and soak for 15 to 30 minutes to allow your body to absorb the benefits.

Store in a sealed glass jar in a cool, dry place.

For maximum freshness and potency, use within 6 months.

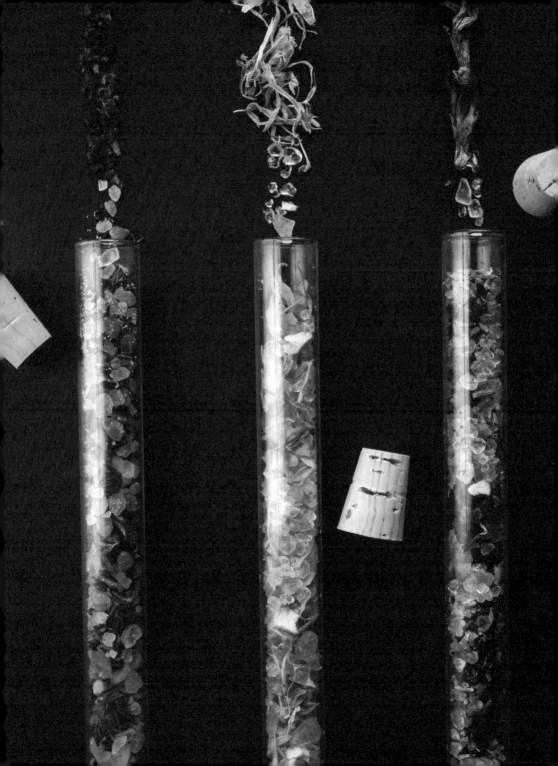

HERBAL ROSE BATH SALTS

Everything's coming up roses with this elegantly scented bath experience. Grounding and relaxing, these salts are excellent for lifting your mood and balancing the system.

MAKES 1½ CUPS

1 cup Himalayan pink salt
½ cup dried rose hips
1 tablespoon dried thyme
10 drops rose essential oil

Mix the ingredients thoroughly in a medium bowl. Add 1½ cups of bath salts to a standard-sized tub while the water is running, to help it dissolve. Fill tub ¾ full of warm water and soak for 15 to 30 minutes to allow your body to absorb the benefits.

Store in a sealed glass jar in a cool, dry place.

For maximum freshness and potency, use within 6 months.

CARESSING CALENDULA BATH SALTS

Escape to a warm, sunny garden with this sweetly scented bath recipe. These herbal salts have the added benefit of soothing and repairing sensitive skin.

MAKES 1½ CUPS

1 cup Epsom salts
½ cup dried calendula
1 tablespoon finely chopped dried orange rind
10 drops chamomile essential oil
5 drops lemon essential oil

Mix the ingredients thoroughly in a medium bowl. Add 1½ cups of bath salts to a standard-sized tub while the water is running, to help it dissolve. Fill tub ¾ full of warm water and soak for 15 to 30 minutes to allow your body to absorb the benefits.

Store in a sealed glass jar in a cool, dry place.

For maximum freshness and potency, use within 6 months.

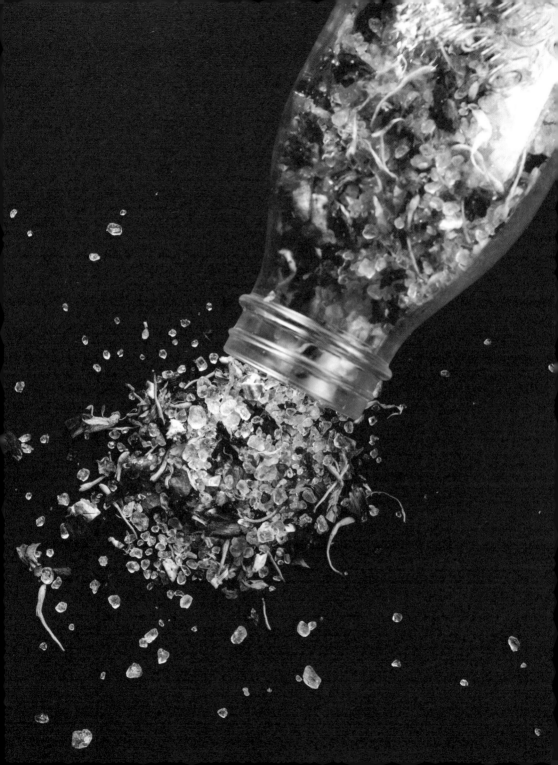

ROCK STAR SALTS

For a tantalizing sensory experience, try this exciting blend.

MAKES 2½ CUPS

2 cups Dead Sea salt
½ cup baking soda
1 teaspoon finely chopped dried grapefruit peel
1 teaspoon dried rose petals
1 teaspoon dried hibiscus flowers
1 teaspoon chopped freeze-dried strawberries
1 teaspoon dried honeysuckle flowers
10 drops bergamot essential oil
10 drops lavender essential oil
10 drops grapefruit essential oil

Mix the ingredients thoroughly in a medium bowl. Add 1½ cups of bath salts to a standard-sized tub while the water is running, to help it dissolve. Fill tub ¾ full of warm water and soak for 15 to 30 minutes to allow your body to absorb the benefits.

Store in a sealed glass jar in a cool, dry place.

For maximum freshness and potency, please use within 6 months.

ESSENTIAL OIL PROPERTIES

+ Bergamot is used to treat stress, depression, anxiety, anorexia, and a number of infections, including skin infections, such as psoriasis and eczema. It is used to stimulate the liver, digestive system, and spleen, and provides an overall lift to those suffering from a general malaise.

+ Chamomile is a powerful calming agent, as well as antibiotic, antiseptic, antidepressant, and an overall mood lifter. The German variety is often better suited to battle inflammation, specifically urinary tract and digestive inflammation. Chamomile also has analgesic properties and can help to eliminate acne.

+ Eucalyptus is a powerful treatment against respiratory issues. In addition, it is used as an antiseptic, antispasmodic, decongestant, diuretic, and stimulant. It also has cooling properties, which gives it deodorizing characteristics; therefore, it helps fight migraines and fevers. This cooling capability also helps with muscle aches and pains.

+ Sweet-smelling jasmine has been known to ease depression and childbirth, in addition to enhancing libido. It's great for respiratory problems, addiction issues, and reducing tension and stress.

+ In addition to providing stress relief, lavender has the following therapeutic properties: antiseptic, antidepressant, anti-inflammatory, decongestant, deodorant, diuretic, and sedative.

+ Lemon oil is a multifaceted essential oil. It helps with everything from skin irritation to digestion to circulation problems. It is a natural immunity booster and can even help reduce cellulite! Lemon oil helps to alleviate headaches and fever, and is a quick mood enhancer.

+ Marjoram aids in anxiety and stress relief, combats fatigue and depression, and alleviates respiratory and circulatory issues.

+ Peppermint oil has a number of therapeutic properties. It is a cooling agent that enhances mood, sharpens focus, combats irritation and redness, alleviates symptoms of congestion, and aids in digestion.

- Rose oil is an ideal essential oil to have on hand. It is good for your skin and helps with a number of illnesses and conditions, such as depression, anxiety, and digestion issues, as well as circulation, heart problems, and respiratory conditions, such as asthma.

- Widely known as a mental stimulant, the antidepressant properties of rosemary oil make it ideal for enhanced memory, focus, and overall brain performance. It also acts as an analgesic, soothing aching, cramping muscles, headaches, and migraines. As an antiseptic it helps with digestive and liver infections. It is great for skin issues as well.

- Sandalwood oil can help mucous membranes of the urinary tract and chest wall. It helps alleviate chest pain. It is also used as a relaxing agent for tension relief. Many practitioners of yoga use sandalwood oil for its calming and sexual properties. It is a hydration aid for the skin, as well as an anti-inflammatory.

- Tea tree oil's healing properties are abundant. Not only is it a natural immunity booster, but it also fights all kinds of infection. It helps heal skin conditions, burns, and cuts, and also works as an insecticide. In addition, it soothes and treats cold sores, respiratory conditions, muscle aches, the flu, athlete's foot, and dandruff. Its uses are vast and its healing power is quick.

- While its calming properties are its most powerful, ylang-ylang oil is also used to soothe headaches, nausea, and skin conditions; stimulate hair growth; reduce high blood pressure; and fight intestinal problems.

✦ ✦ ✦ ✦

BEAUTY NOTE

Essential oils are volatile liquids distilled from plants. They must be purely distilled to protect their chemical constituents, which are affected by soil conditions, climate, temperature, harvest. Always choose certified, pure, therapeutic-grade oils.

✦ ✦ ✦ ✦

STRAWBERRY LOVE BATH BOMBS

As fun as commercial bath bombs can be, they are often infused with neurotoxic ingredients that may interfere with the liver's ability to detoxify properly. The good news is that they are actually quite simple to replicate at home, safely, using all-natural ingredients.

MAKES 6 TO 8 BOMBS

2 cups baking soda
1 cup citric acid
¼ cup chopped freeze-dried strawberries
10 drops rose essential oil (optional)
Witch hazel

Select your preferred molds. Standard size (2-by-1¼ inches) silicone muffin molds or baking tins with liners will allow for easy product removal.

Place the baking soda and citric acid in a large, nonreactive bowl and mix well. Add the strawberries and the essential oil, if using, and mix, using your hands.

Spray the mixture with five spritzes of witch hazel and mix by hand. Add several more spritzes over the entire surface of the mixture, until it reaches a damp, sandlike consistency that holds together. Working quickly, firmly press the mixture into your designated molds. Let sit in a cool, dry spot for a few hours, then remove from the molds.

To use: Drop one bomb into a tub of warm water, hop in, and get fizzy with it!

Store in a sealed container in a cool, dry place. For maximum freshness and potency, please use within 6 months.

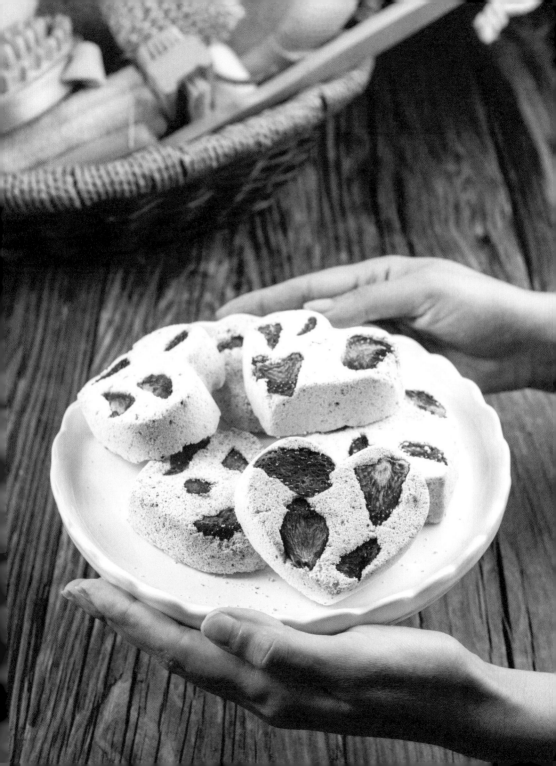

YOU'RE THE BOMB AROMATHERAPY SHOWER TABLETS

You can harness the healing benefits of steam bathing in your own shower by making these aromatherapy shower steamers. These small tablets that you place in your tub or stall at the far end of your shower, out of the stream of water, will fizz, allowing the essential oils to float up into the steam, giving you a therapeutic experience that can help with congestion, soothe nerves, and uplift your spirits. You can customize your experience by varying the essential oils you use.

MAKES 4 TABLETS OR 8 OUNCES

1 cup baking soda
1 tablespoon arrowroot flour
⅓ cup water
5 drops eucalyptus essential oil
5 drops lavender essential oil
5 drops rosemary essential oil
5 drops lemon essential oil

Select your preferred molds. Silicone or lined molds work best. Mix together the baking soda and arrowroot in a medium bowl and slowly add the water.

Pour this mixture into your designated molds. Let set overnight. Once set, add the essential oils.

To use: Drop one tablet into your tub or shower stall, away from the stream of water, and sprinkle a little bit of water on the tablet to activate it. Breathe in the aromatherapy.

Store in a sealed container in a cool, dry place. For maximum freshness and potency, please use within 6 months.

✦ ✦ ✦ ✦

APOTHECARY TIP

If you prefer not to make bombs, combine the baking soda with the essential oils and transfer the dry mixture to a lidded glass jar. To use, sprinkle 1 to 2 tablespoons of the powder on the bottom of your tub or shower stall and turn on the hot water. Alternatively, the powder can be added to bathwater.

✦ ✦ ✦ ✦

Brush Your Way to Healthy Skin

Dry brushing is a lovely self-care technique that encourages the circulation of lymph, a detoxifying, nutrient-delivering fluid that flows just beneath the skin. To get your lymph flowing and improving circulation and the health of your skin, brush your naked body with a stiff-bristled body brush, working from your feet up, using circular strokes in the direction of your heart. Dry brush at least once a week, after bathing, for softer, healthier skin.

CHAI EXFOLIATING LOTION BARS

These intoxicating chai-infused lotion bars do double duty, both exfoliating and moisturizing your skin. The surprising addition of the mighty chia seed, packed with omega-3 fatty acids, also helps fight free radicals and repair damaged skin.

MAKES 6 TO 8 BARS

Grapeseed oil or any neutral natural oil, for molds
½ cup cocoa butter
¼ cup shea butter
¼ cup almond meal
¼ cup chia seeds
1 teaspoon ground cardamom
1 teaspoon ground cinnamon
1 teaspoon black tea leaves
1 teaspoon pure vanilla extract

Grease your preferred molds with oil. Standard size (2-by-1¼ inches) silicone muffin molds or baking tins with liners will allow for easy removal.

Melt the cocoa butter and shea butter in a double boiler or a heat-safe bowl perched over a saucepan of simmering water. Remove from the heat and stir in the almond meal, chia seeds, cardamom, cinnamon, tea leaves, and vanilla. Pour the mixture into your molds. Allow to fully cool and settle before removing.

To use: Moisten your skin under the shower and rub the bar all over your body for a deeply moisturizing and exfoliating experience.

Store in a sealed container in a cool, dark place. For maximum freshness and potency, please use within 6 months.

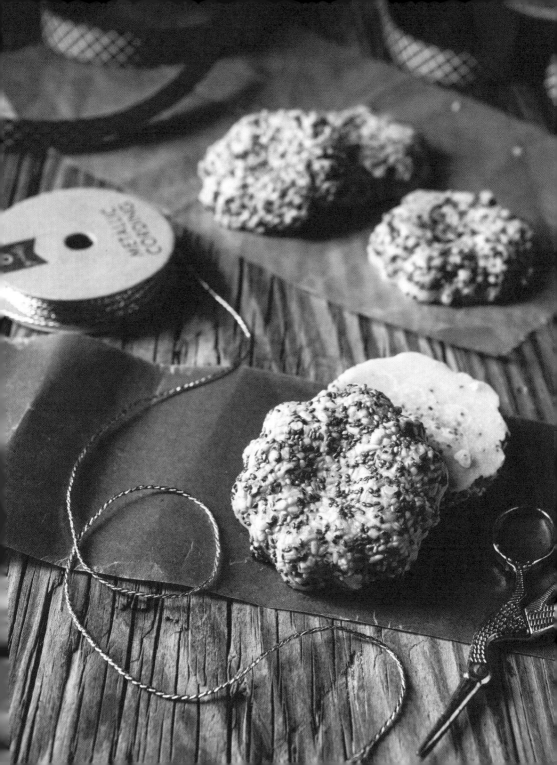

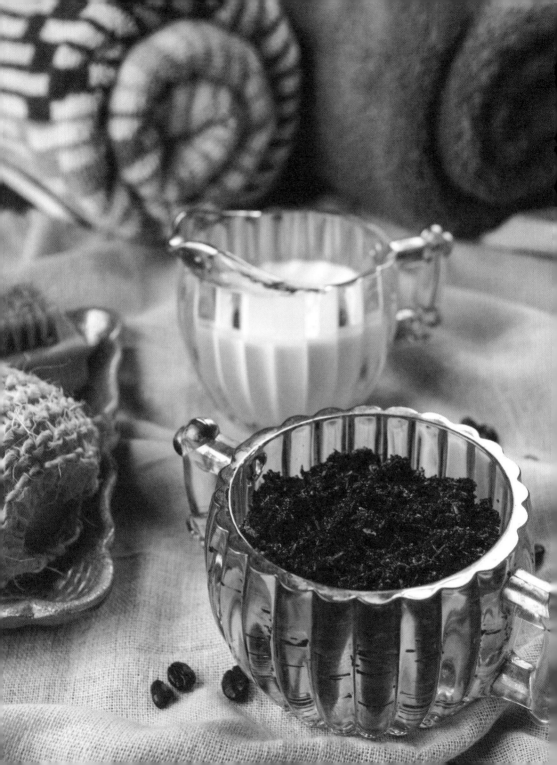

COFFEE BODY SCRUB

Revive your tired skin with this invigorating caffeinated exfoliator. The antioxidant-rich coffee grounds and warming cinnamon stimulate blood flow, while the skin-soothing coconut oil moisturizes, resulting in a scrub that will give you smoother, firmer skin instantly.

MAKES 1 CUP

½ cup brewed coffee grounds
1 tablespoon ground cinnamon
¼ cup sugar
2 teaspoons pure vanilla extract
¼ cup melted coconut oil

Mix together the coffee grounds, cinnamon, sugar, vanilla, and melted oil in a small bowl to create a spreadable paste. Transfer to a lidded glass jar.

To use: While standing in the shower, scrub the exfoliating mixture all over your body, paying extra attention to possible problem areas. Rinse well.

Store in its sealed glass jar in the refrigerator. For maximum freshness and potency, please use within 6 months.

✦ ✦ ✦ ✦

BEAUTY NOTE

For a truly pampering experience, pour 1 cup of room-temperature pure coconut milk all over your body after applying the scrub. Luxuriate before rinsing off the scrub with warm water.

✦ ✦ ✦ ✦

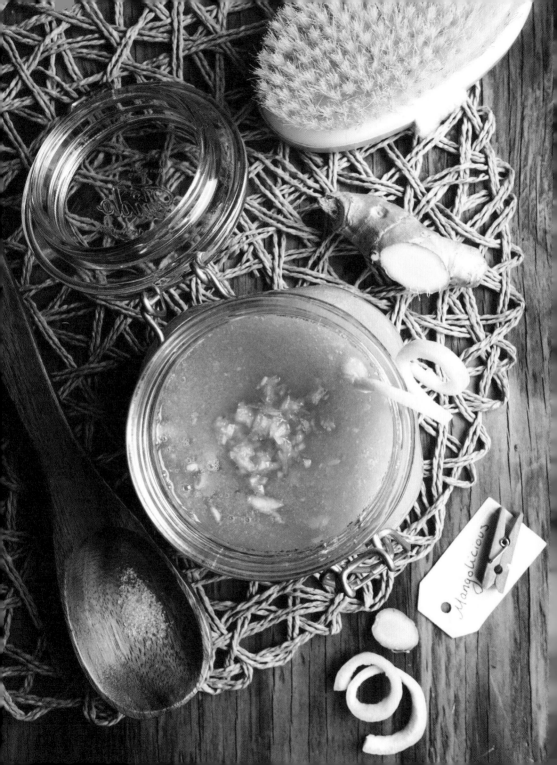

LUSCIOUS MANGO
BODY POLISH

Immerse your skin in a lush tropical experience with this sweet, aromatic polish. Vitamin A–rich mango, in collaboration with the spicy ginger and fresh lemon, works gently to reveal the softest skin.

MAKES 2½ CUPS

2 cups sugar (I used coconut sugar)
1 tablespoon lemon zest
2 teaspoons ground ginger
1 cup mango puree
2 tablespoons grapeseed oil

Combine the sugar, lemon zest, ginger, and mango puree in a bowl and mix thoroughly. Transfer to a lidded glass jar.

To use: While in the shower, scrub the mixture into your skin, using circular motions, paying special attention to your elbows, knees, and rough spots.

Store in its sealed glass container in the refrigerator. For maximum freshness and potency, please use within 6 months.

DETOXIFYING CHARCOAL BODY SCRUB

This no-nonsense body scrub detoxifies your body at the cellular level. Activated charcoal works to draw out dirt, toxins, and impurities, while the tea tree oil helps protect against odor, blemishes, and infections.

MAKES 1 CUP

1 cup sea salt
2 tablespoons grapeseed oil
Contents of 5 activated charcoal capsules, or 1 tablespoon charcoal powder
10 drops tea tree oil (optional)

Place the salt, oil, and activated charcoal in a bowl and mix until fully combined. Add the tea tree oil, if using. Transfer to a lidded glass jar.

To use: Use in the shower by massaging onto wet skin, using circular motions. Rinse under warm water.

Store in its sealed glass jar in the refrigerator. For maximum freshness and potency, please use within 6 months.

✦ ✦ ✦ ✦

APOTHECARY TIP

To avoid staining, take care to rinse away any charcoal residue from your tub or shower stall directly after use.

✦ ✦ ✦ ✦

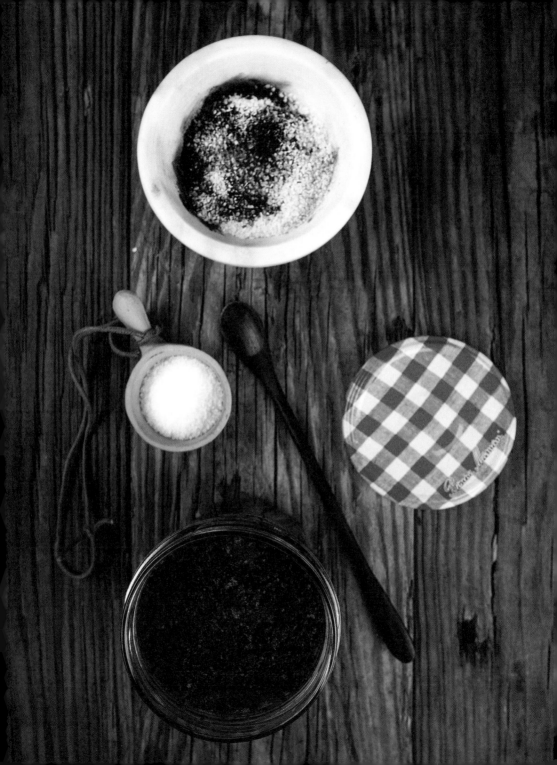

SEA MUD FIRMING BODY WRAP

Take your homemade body treatment to the next level with this ocean botanical, herb, and clay wrap. This clarifying and detoxifying wrap will tone every inch of your body while stimulating your lymphatic system.

MAKES I TREATMENT

2 tablespoons dried sage leaves
½ cup boiling water
½ cup aloe vera water
¼ cup powdered kelp
¼ cup French green clay
Essential oils (optional)

Steep the sage in the boiling water for 20 minutes. Strain the infusion into a nonmetal bowl and add the aloe water and powdered kelp. Mix in the clay, using a nonmetal spoon, and stir until a smooth paste is achieved. Add essential oils, if using.

To use: While standing in an empty tub, spread the mixture carefully all over your body and wrap each section in plastic wrap. Cover up in a towel and relax in the tub for 30 minutes.

Remove the towel and plastic wrap and rinse off the mud with warm water.

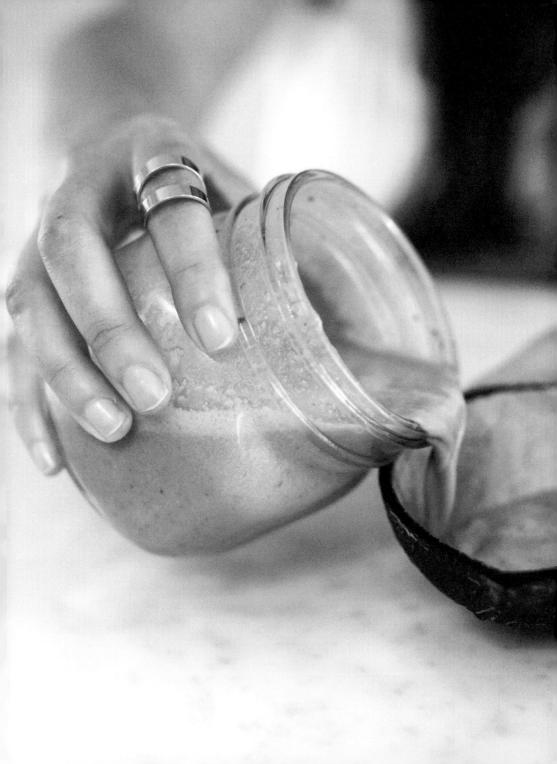

ORANGE BLOSSOM AND LEMON BALM BODY LOTION

Lemon balm, an herb also known as Melissa, has been used in traditional medicine to treat a number of health concerns, including insomnia, anxiety, and migraines.

Its springtime aroma is both uplifting and soothing, while its antiviral and antimicrobial properties make it a valued plant to use in topical applications. It can help reduce swelling, relieve pain, and heal wounds faster. Not bad properties to infuse your body lotion with.

MAKES 1½ CUPS

¾ cup Lemon Balm–Infused Oil (page 136)
3 tablespoons vegetable wax
¾ cup orange blossom water
Aloe

Melt together the infused oil and wax in a double boiler or a heat-safe bowl perched over a saucepan of simmering water. Remove from the heat and let cool. Slowly add the orange blossom water while whisking continuously, until a creamy consistency is achieved. Pour the lotion into a lidded glass jar.

To use: Pour a small amount into the palm of your hand and blend into your skin.

Store in its sealed glass jar in a cool, dark place. For maximum freshness and potency, please use within 6 months.

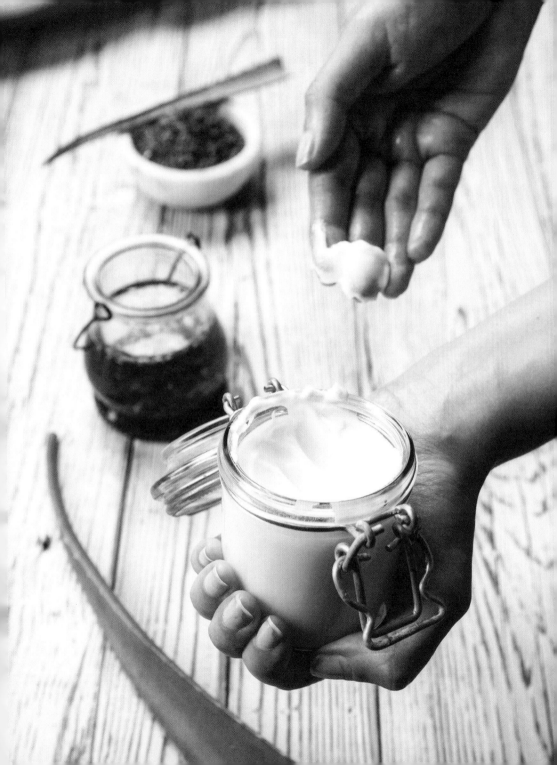

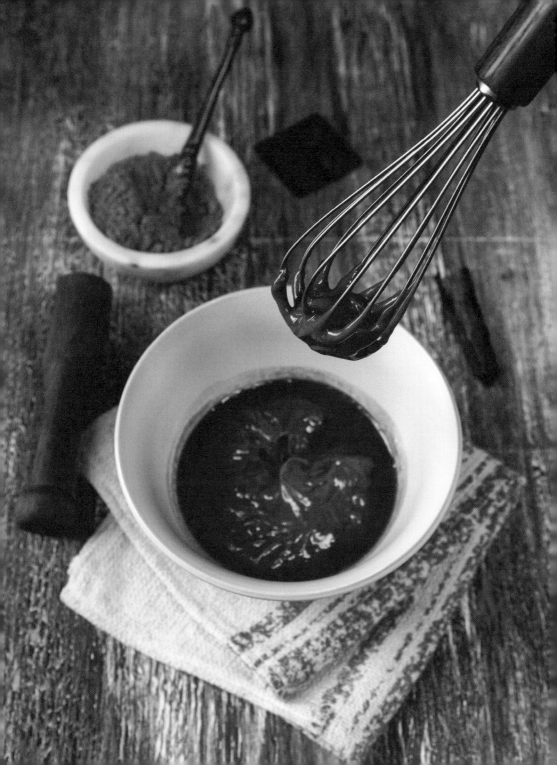

CHOCOLATE SOUFFLÉ BODY BUTTER

Admit it! At some point in your life, you've dreamed of slathering yourself in chocolate. I know I have! Now you can safely indulge in the fantasy without making a mess. This indulgent, antioxidant-rich body butter is everything. I can't get enough.

MAKES I CUP

½ cup cocoa butter
½ cup coconut oil
2 tablespoons cacao powder
1 teaspoon pure vanilla extract

Melt the cocoa butter and coconut oil in a double boiler or a heat-safe bowl perched over a saucepan of simmering water. Remove from the heat and allow to cool. Stir in the cacao powder and vanilla. Let chill in the refrigerator for 30 minutes, then blend the butter, using a whisk, until fluffy. Transfer to a lidded glass jar.

To use: Smooth the creamy butter onto your skin for a moisturizing treat.

Store in a sealed glass jar in a cool, dry spot. For maximum freshness and potency, please use within 6 months.

WARMING VANILLA BODY OIL

Sultry and exotic, this infused body oil pampers you with its warm spices. The perfect moisturizer for cold winter mornings.

MAKES I CUP

Water
1 cup sesame oil
1 teaspoon grated fresh ginger
1 teaspoon black peppercorns
1 teaspoon cardamom pods
1 vanilla bean

Bring 2 inches of water to a boil in a small saucepan and lower the heat to low. Place a heat-safe glass bowl inside the saucepan and add the sesame oil. Gently heat the oil and add the ginger, peppercorns, and cardamom pods. Then cut open the vanilla bean and scrape the contents into the mixture, adding the empty pods as well.

Continue to heat on low for 40 minutes, taking care not to boil the oil mixture. Remove from the heat and allow to cool. Strain out the solids, using a mesh strainer, and transfer to a lidded glass bottle.

To use: Pour a small amount of oil in your palm and smooth onto your skin for a warming moisturizer.

Store in its sealed glass bottle in a cool, dry spot. For maximum freshness and potency, please use within 6 months.

❖ ❖ ❖ ❖

APOTHECARY TIP

For more information on oil infusions, please review page 208.

❖ ❖ ❖ ❖

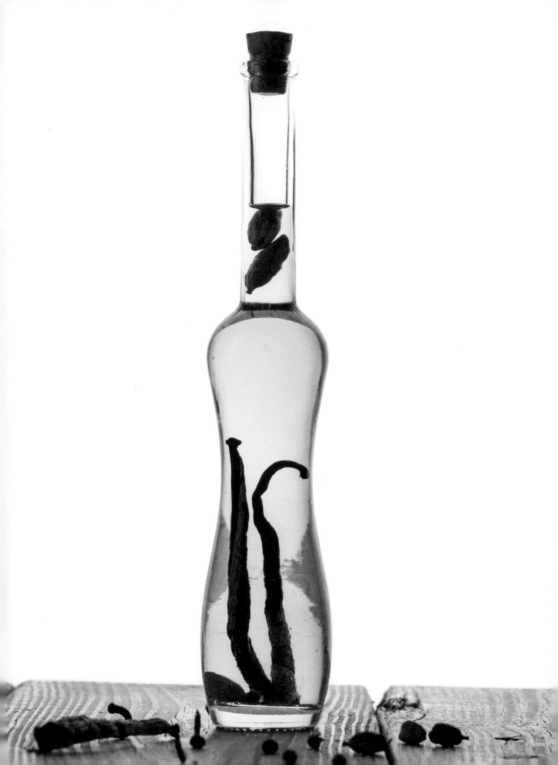

PERFUME BALM

MAKES I OUNCE

1 tablespoon vegetable wax
1 tablespoon grapeseed oil
8 drops essential oil of your choice

Gently melt the wax and oil in a heat-resistant container or saucepan. Remove from the heat and stir in the essential oil. Transfer to a lidded tin or small glass container. Allow the mixture to cool completely before closing the lid.

To use: Rub the perfume on your pulse points and wherever else you like.

Store in its sealed container in a cool, dry spot. For maximum freshness and potency, please use within 6 months.

If you prefer an oil perfume instead of a solid, simply omit the wax from the Perfume Balm recipe.

In either case, here are a few blends that work incredibly well together:

FRUITY: 2 drops each of peach, sweet orange, grapefruit, and chamomile essential oils

SPICY: 2 drops each of clove, sandalwood, cinnamon, rose, and bergamot essential oils

EXOTIC: 4 drops of pure vanilla extract plus 2 drops each of ylang-ylang, jasmine, and black pepper essential oils

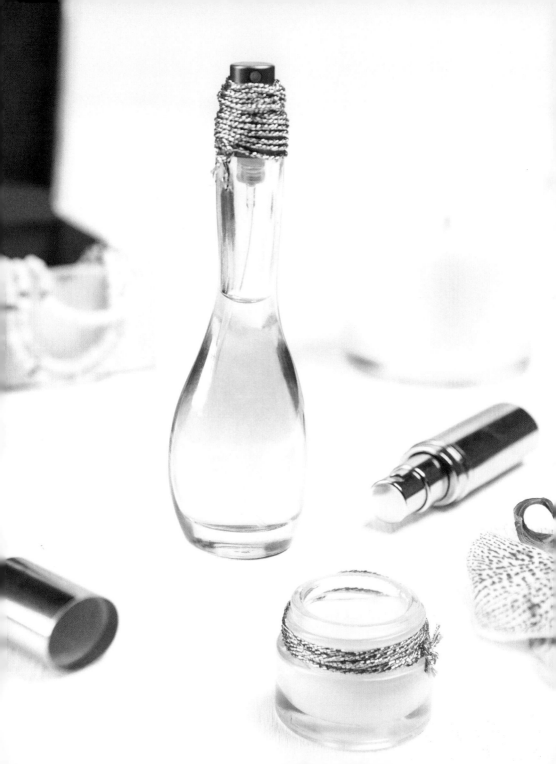

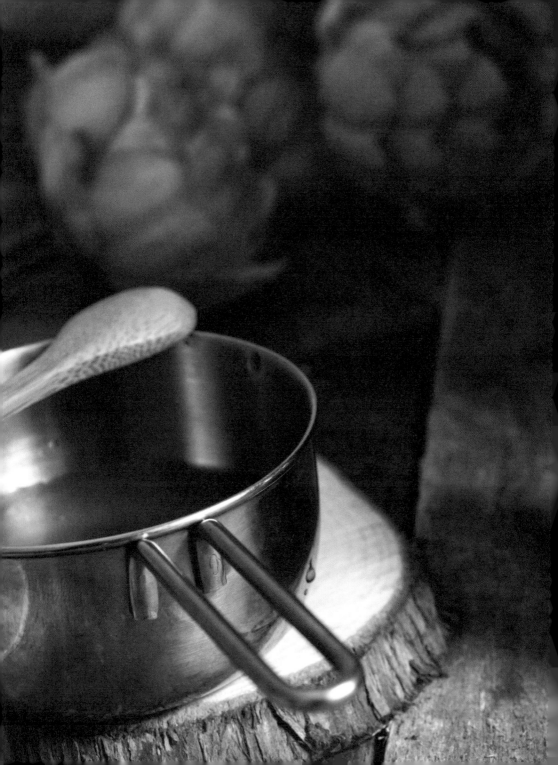

SENSUAL MASSAGE OIL

Ylang-ylang and jasmine essential oils are stimulants and aphrodisiacs that uplift your mood while soothing your body. These exotic oils blend especially well together.

MAKES ½ CUP

½ cup sweet almond oil
8 drops ylang-ylang essential oil
8 drops sweet orange essential oil
8 drops jasmine essential oil

Mix together in a lidded glass container.

Store in its sealed glass container in a cool, dry spot. For maximum freshness and potency, please use within 6 months.

How to Give a Great Massage

- *Choose a firm, steady surface: a massage table, yoga mat, or quilts on the floor will do.*

- *Set the mood. Create a relaxing environment with candlelight, soft music, and relaxing essential oils.*

- *Tune in to your partner's needs. Adjust your pressure and concentrate on possible problem areas.*

- *Keep your strokes smooth and flowing, always going in the direction of the heart, just like the flow of the valves in your veins.*

- *Savor the moment and allow your partner to linger and relax after the massage.*

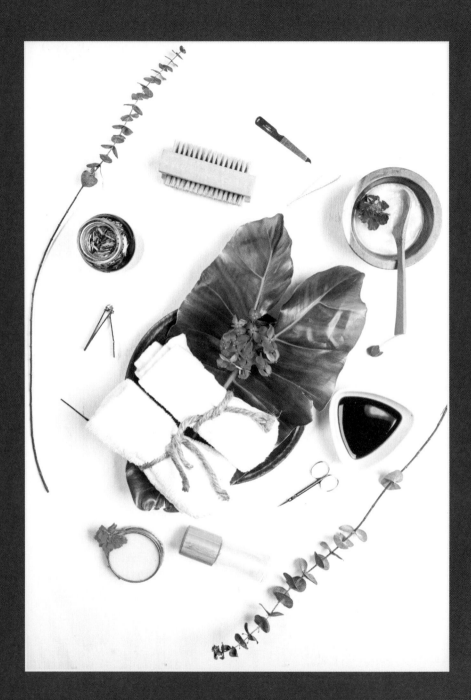

HAND AND FOOT CARE

No beauty care regimen is complete without the proper care of our hands and feet. The most hardworking parts of our bodies—our extremities—need extra loving care. Treating them to a simple regimen of daily care will keep them healthy and happy for years to come. Here are some recipes to get you started.

Comfrey and Lemon Balm All-Purpose Healing Salve

Moisturizing Hand Sanitizer

Hand and Foot Scrub

Molasses Nail-Strengthening and Conditioning Soak

Mustard Foot Soak

Minty Fresh Foot Powder

COMFREY AND LEMON BALM ALL-PURPOSE HEALING SALVE

This magical salve is infused with the special healing abilities of the delicate purple blossom comfrey. Use it to soften overworked hands and feet, and try it on scrapes, burns, and blemishes to truly experience its healing powers.

MAKES 8 OUNCES

COMFREY AND LEMON BALM–INFUSED OLIVE OIL
¼ cup dried comfrey leaves
¼ cup dried lemon balm
1 cup olive oil

FOR THE SALVE
2 teaspoons vegetable wax
2 tablespoons shea butter
1 cup comfrey and lemon balm–infused olive oil
1 teaspoon vitamin E oil
10 drops lemon balm essential oil (optional)

To prepare the comfrey and lemon balm–infused olive oil, follow the instructions on page 208, or for a quick version, do the following:

On the lowest setting on your stove, place the comfrey leaves, lemon balm, and oil in a double boiler and cover with a tightly fitting lid. Bring the water in the lower pan to a simmer and allow the oil to heat for 20 to 30 minutes, being careful not to cook the flowers.

Decant the infused oil through cheesecloth into a glass jar.

To make the salve, melt the wax and shea butter in a double boiler or a heat-safe bowl perched over a saucepan of simmering water. Once the ingredients have melted, remove from the heat. Add the infused oil, vitamin E, and essential oil, if using. Transfer to a lidded tin or glass jar and let set, then seal.

Store in its sealed container in a cool, dry place. For maximum freshness and potency, please use within 6 months.

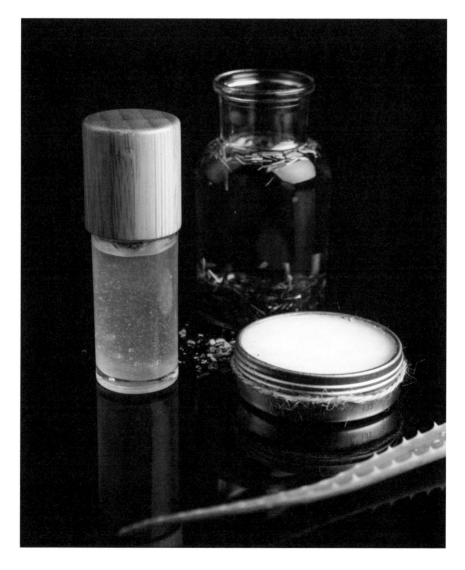

MOISTURIZING HAND SANITIZER

Replace your chemical-laden sanitizer with this all-natural solution for a clean, moisturizing experience.

MAKES 1½ OUNCES

1 tablespoon witch hazel
2 tablespoons aloe vera gel
5 drops grapefruit essential oil (optional)
5 drops lavender essential oil (optional)

Mix together the witch hazel and aloe vera gel in a lidded 2-ounce glass bottle. Using an eyedropper, add the essential oils, if using. Close the lid and shake the bottle until the ingredients are well blended.

To use: Dispense a small amount into your palm and rub all over your hands. Carry with you to fight germs on the go.

Store in its sealed glass bottle. For maximum freshness and potency, please use within 1 month.

HAND AND FOOT SCRUB

This scrub, specially formulated to exfoliate the skin on your hands and feet, will leave you feeling soft and smooth from hand to toe.

MAKES 1 TREATMENT

2 tablespoons baking soda
2 teaspoons sesame oil
2 teaspoons fresh lemon juice

Stir together all the ingredients in a small bowl to create a thick, spreadable paste.

To use: Apply the mixture immediately to dry hands and feet and rub them well, making sure to massage paste in between fingers and toes, around nails and cuticles, and on the back of hands and feet. Allow to penetrate for an additional 5 minutes and rinse with warm water.

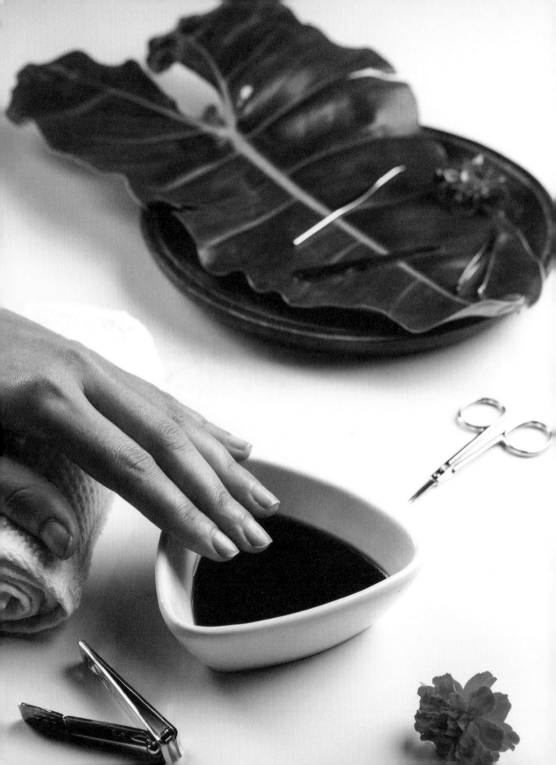

MOLASSES NAIL-STRENGTHENING AND CONDITIONING SOAK

Molasses is made from the juice of fresh sugarcane. It is an excellent humectant that can help restore lost moisture to skin and nails, while its high mineral content strengthens and beautifies nails. Use this simple soak to soften cuticles and condition nails before a manicure.

MAKES 1 TREATMENT

¼ cup warm water
2 tablespoons molasses

Mix together the water and molasses in a small bowl, stirring well.

To use: Immediately soak your nails in the solution for 15 to 20 minutes.

✦ ✦ ✦ ✦

BEAUTY NOTE

To ensure bright, healthy nails, add a tablespoon of fresh lemon juice to the solution.

✦ ✦ ✦ ✦

MUSTARD FOOT SOAK

A hot mustard bath helps open up the pores, allowing toxins and impurities to slip away while relieving stress and muscle soreness. Use as a foot soak or as a bath to relieve tired muscles.

MAKES 1 BATH OR 6 FOOT SOAKS

2 tablespoons baking soda
2 tablespoons Epsom salts
2 tablespoons dry ground mustard
1 tablespoon ground turmeric
2 drops eucalyptus essential oil

Mix together all the ingredients in a small bowl. Transfer to a lidded glass container if planning to use for foot soaks.

To use: For a bath, add to running bathwater. For a footbath, add 1 tablespoon of the mixture to a basin of hot water and soak your feet for 15 minutes.

Store in its sealed glass container in a cool, dry place. For maximum freshness and potency, please use within 6 months.

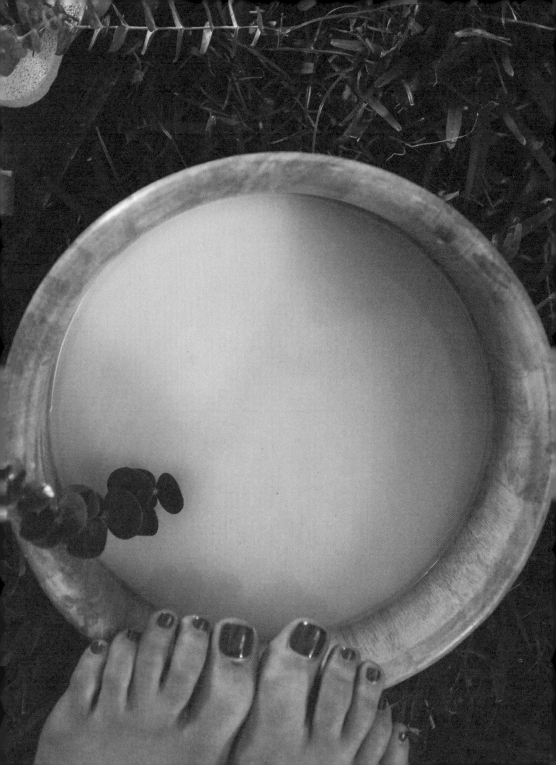

MINTY FRESH FOOT POWDER

This refreshing and stimulating powder will keep moisture away. A perfect choice to sprinkle in your shoes on hot summer days. Works equally well as an all-body deodorizer to use before and after exercise.

MAKES 1 CUP

¼ cup dried peppermint
½ cup baking soda
½ cup white clay
20 drops lemon and/or peppermint essential oil

Place the dried mint in a spice or coffee grinder and grind into a fine powder. Transfer to a small bowl and mix with the clay and baking soda. Add the essential oil and mix again. Allow the oil to be absorbed, then transfer to a lidded glass jar.

To use: Apply as you would any foot or body powder. This is especially effective for keeping feet and underarms dry.

Store in its sealed glass jar. For maximum freshness and potency, please use within 6 months.

Tips for Healthy Hands and Feet

- *Your trusty face and body mask works wonders on your hands and feet as well. Apply using the same instructions as for your face or body.*

  - *Soak your fingertips and toes, using the Molasses Nail-Strengthening and Conditioning Soak (page 141).*

- *Massage your hands and feet with cream or body oil and wrap in plastic wrap, or cotton gloves and socks, for 30 minutes or overnight.*

  - *Polish your nails by rubbing oil on them and buffing them to increase circulation.*

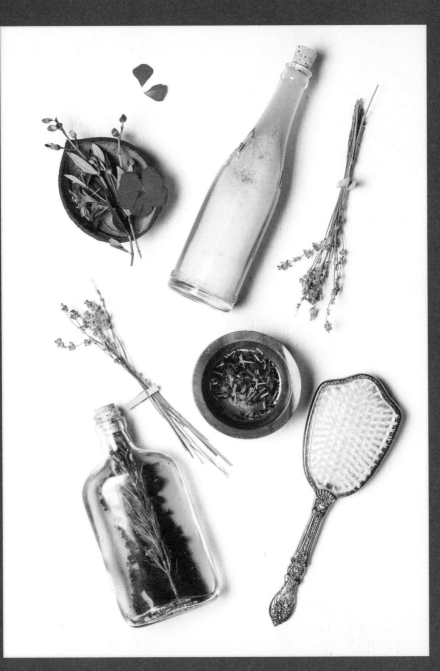

HAIR CARE

The following hair care recipes are gentle on your hair and scalp. It might require a period of adjustment to reverse the damage of overwashing and styling, but these simple recipes will keep your hair strong, shiny, and soft in no time.

Calendula Blossom Shampoo

Natural Dry Shampoo

Herbal Hair Rinse

Rosemary Hot Oil Treatment

Deep Hair Conditioner

Pumpkin Spice and Molasses Scalp Treatment

Mint and Avocado Hair Repair Mask

Split End Healing Serum

Hair Frizz Tamer Spray

Beach Day Hair Spray

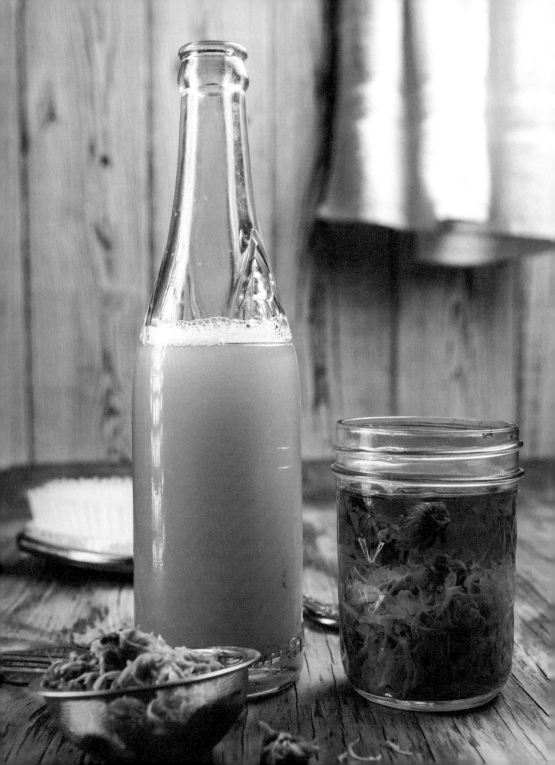

CALENDULA BLOSSOM SHAMPOO

This gentle, effective hair wash, made with the unique antioxidant compounds found in the calendula blossom, helps restore health and vitality to your hair and scalp.

MAKES 2 CUPS

2 cups distilled water
¼ cup dried calendula blossoms
¼ cup Castile soap
2 tablespoons glycerin
5 drops lavender essential oils (optional)
5 drops rosemary essential oils (optional)
5 drops chamomile essential oils (optional)

Place the calendula blossoms in a heatproof medium bowl. Bring the distilled water to a boil and pour over the calendula. Allow to steep for 20 minutes, strain, and allow to cool. Add the rest of the ingredients and stir well. Decant into a lidded glass bottle.

To use: Integrate into your routine as your primary hair cleanser.

Store in its sealed glass bottle. For maximum freshness and potency, please use within 1 month.

NATURAL DRY SHAMPOO

Revitalize and refresh hair with a natural dry shampoo you can feel good about. You'll love these volumizing and color-specific options.

MAKES 1 APPLICATION

FOR LIGHT HAIR
1 tablespoon rolled oats
¼ cup arrowroot flour

FOR DARK HAIR
1 tablespoon rolled oats
2 tablespoons raw cacao powder

Grind the oats in a nut or coffee grinder to create a fine powder.

Combine the oat powder with the other ingredients and mix thoroughly. Place in a large-holed shaker spice jar with a tight-fitting lid.

To use: Sprinkle the powder onto the roots of dry hair and brush through your locks.

Store in its sealed glass jar. For maximum freshness and potency, please use within 1 year.

When to Wash

No matter what your hair care routine consists of, chances are, you're washing your hair far too often. Traditional shampoo strips your hair of its natural oils and disturbs the natural balance needed for healthy hair growth. The oil on your scalp is not the enemy. In fact, it helps keep the rest of your hair healthy and well moisturized, if you let it. Aim to wash your hair every seven to ten days.

To ease the transition, use a natural-bristle hairbrush that soaks up hair oils, allowing you to distribute the oils evenly throughout your hair all the way from the roots to the ends.

If your head sweats during exercise, you can rinse your hair with cool water, using minimal scrubbing, to lift away dirt and sweat but not the oils, between your weekly washes.

Use only natural shampoos and conditioners without harsh lathering agents such as sulfates, and avoid using any products containing silicone.

And finally, you can use a gentle, nonirritating, and nondrying dry shampoo, such as the Natural Dry Shampoo, to keep you going between washes.

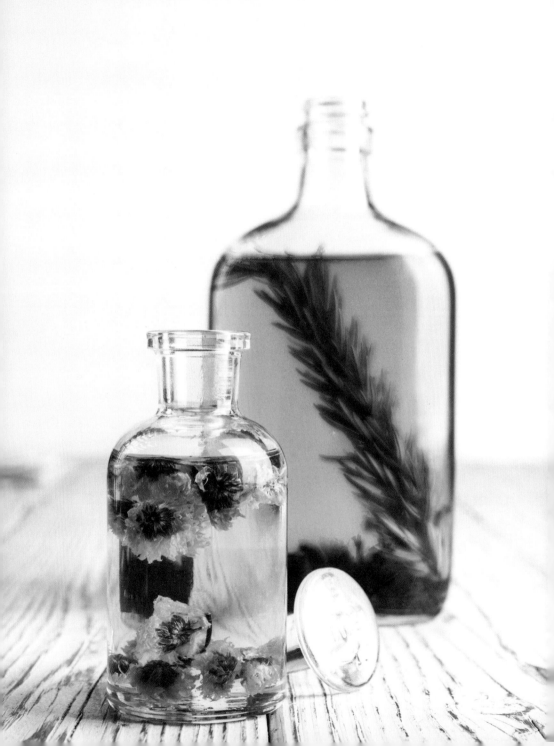

HERBAL HAIR RINSE

Eliminate buildup and restore shine with this effective herbal hair rinse.

Nettle's antioxidant, antimicrobial, and astringent properties strengthen hair and restore its and your scalp's natural pH balance.

MAKES I RINSE

2 cups distilled water
1 teaspoon green tea leaves, or 2 tea bags
1 tablespoon dried nettles
1 tablespoon dried rosemary
2 tablespoons raw apple cider vinegar

About an hour before you plan to wash your hair, bring the distilled water to a boil in a large pot. Add the green tea, nettles, and rosemary. Remove from the heat, cover with a lid, and allow to cool completely, about 1 hour. Strain and discard the solids. Add the vinegar.

To use: Shampoo your hair as normal, then follow with the herbal rinse. Allow it to fully absorb without rinsing it out. Wrap your hair in a towel and dry as usual.

ROSEMARY HOT OIL TREATMENT

Heating this deeply nourishing oil infusion allows nutrients to penetrate into the hair shaft, giving hair extra luster.

MAKES I TREATMENT

ROSEMARY-INFUSED OLIVE OIL
2 tablespoons dried rosemary
6 tablespoons olive oil

FOR THE TREATMENT
5 tablespoons rosemary-infused olive oil
3 drops rosemary essential oil (optional)
3 drops cedarwood essential oil (optional)

About 30 minutes before you plan to treat your hair, prepare the oil infusion, following the instructions on page 208, or use the following quick method:

Place the rosemary and olive oil in a double boiler and cover with a tightly fitting lid. Over the lowest possible heat, bring the water in the lower pot to a simmer and allow the oil to heat for 20 to 30 minutes, taking care not to burn the herbs. Decant your oil through cheesecloth into a glass jar.

Let cool until the oil is lukewarm, then add the essential oil, if using.

To use: Work the mixture into your scalp and comb to saturate the strands. Wrap your hair with a warm, wet towel and allow the oil to permeate your hair. Rinse and wash as usual.

DEEP HAIR CONDITIONER

This deeply moisturizing hair treatment with argan oil helps control frizz, repairs split ends, and soothes dry scalp. The addition of precious carrot oil, rich in vitamins and silica, helps renew hair growth and straightens hair follicles.

MAKES 2 OUNCES

2 tablespoons coconut oil
1 tablespoon shea butter
1 teaspoon argan oil
1 teaspoon carrot seed oil

Heat the coconut oil and shea butter in a heat-safe bowl or saucepan over gentle heat until fully melted. Remove from the heat, let cool, and add the argan and carrot seed oils. Stir well, refrigerate for 20 minutes, then whisk until frothy. Transfer to a lidded glass jar.

To use: Comb the conditioner through your hair and scalp and cover with a shower cap. Leave on for 30 minutes and rinse thoroughly.

Store in its sealed glass jar in a cool, dry place. For maximum freshness and potency, please use within 3 months.

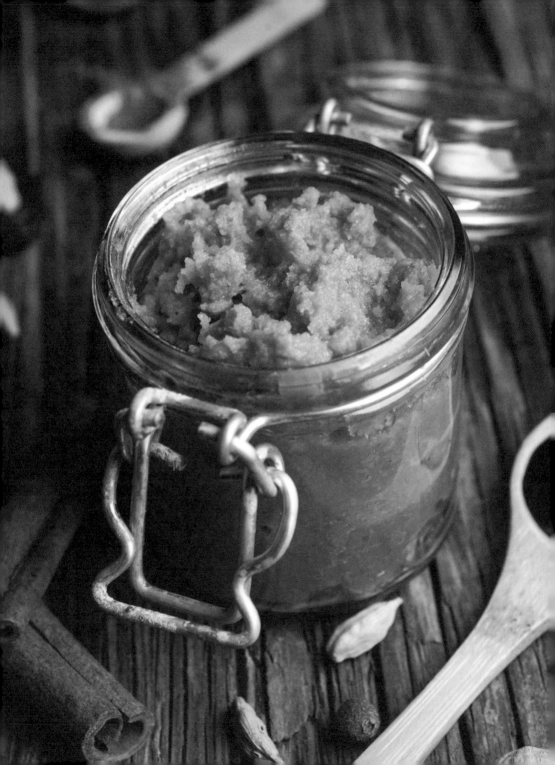

PUMPKIN SPICE AND MOLASSES SCALP TREATMENT

For your hair to grow thick and strong, start with a healthy scalp. This mineral-rich treatment, made with fresh pumpkin, nourishes the scalp, while the antioxidants promote hair growth and strengthen hair follicles.

MAKES 1 TREATMENT

½ cup canned or fresh pure pumpkin puree
2 tablespoons coconut oil
1 tablespoon molasses
1 teaspoon mixed ground nutmeg, cinnamon, and cloves (optional)

Immediately before use, mix all the ingredients together in a small bowl until well blended.

To use: Apply the mixture to your hair, cover with a shower cap, and allow the mixture to penetrate your scalp for 15 to 20 minutes. Rinse thoroughly.

MINT AND AVOCADO HAIR REPAIR MASK

This deep-conditioning hair mask, full of vitamins C, E, and K and rich proteins and fats from the avocado, will envelop the most damaged hair with nourishing properties; the peppermint tea invigorates the scalp, leaving you with luscious, moisturized locks and a fresh, clean feeling.

MAKES 1 TREATMENT

¼ cup peppermint tea leaves
¼ cup boiling water
1 avocado
1 tablespoon avocado oil
5 drops peppermint essential oil (optional)

Place the peppermint tea leaves in a small heatproof bowl. Pour the boiling water over the mint leaves. Allow to infuse for 15 minutes, let cool, and strain.

Pit, peel, and mash the avocado in a separate small bowl, add the avocado oil, peppermint tea, and essential oil, if using, and mix well.

To use: Massage into your hair, concentrating on the ends, and allow to permeate for 20 minutes. Rinse thoroughly.

For maximum freshness and potency, use immediately.

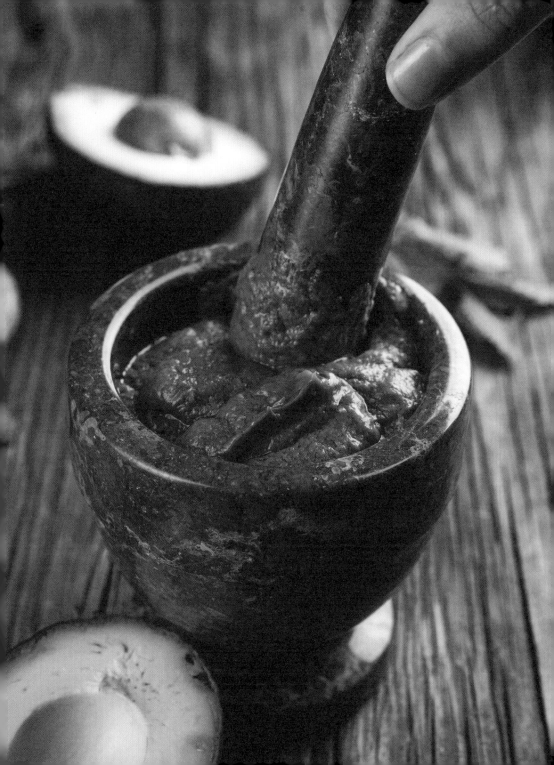

SPLIT END HEALING SERUM

Mend and prevent split ends with this magical serum that coats and nourishes dry hair.

MAKES 1 OR 2 TREATMENTS

2 tablespoons coconut oil
2 teaspoons neem oil
2 teaspoons carrot seed oil
10 drops rosemary essential oil (optional)

Mix together all the ingredients in a lidded glass jar.

To use: Coat the hair with the oil and massage it into your scalp and ends. Leave on for 20 to 30 minutes. Rinse thoroughly and shampoo as usual.

Store in its sealed glass jar in a cool, dry place. For maximum freshness and potency, please use within 3 months.

HAIR FRIZZ TAMER SPRAY

Tame frizz and fly-aways with this light, silky spray.

MAKES 5 OUNCES

¼ cup water
¼ cup rose water
1 teaspoon glycerin
2 tablespoons aloe vera gel

Mix together all the ingredients in a small bowl until well blended, then transfer to a spray bottle.

To use: Shake the bottle vigorously, then spritz the mixture on wet or dry hair to hydrate the hair shafts and smooth frizz.

Store in its spray bottle. For maximum freshness and potency, please use within 3 months.

BEACH DAY HAIR SPRAY

Those soft beachy waves you get after a day by the ocean? The irresistible seaside texture minus the sand and sun are yours in this simple homemade formula.

MAKES 9 OUNCES

1 cup distilled water
1 tablespoon sea salt
1 teaspoon coconut oil
1 teaspoon aloe vera gel

Place all the ingredients in a spray bottle and gently shake to combine.

To use: Spray onto damp or dry hair to add a day-at-the-beach texture to your locks.

Store in its bottle in a cool, dark place. For maximum freshness and potency, please use within 3 months.

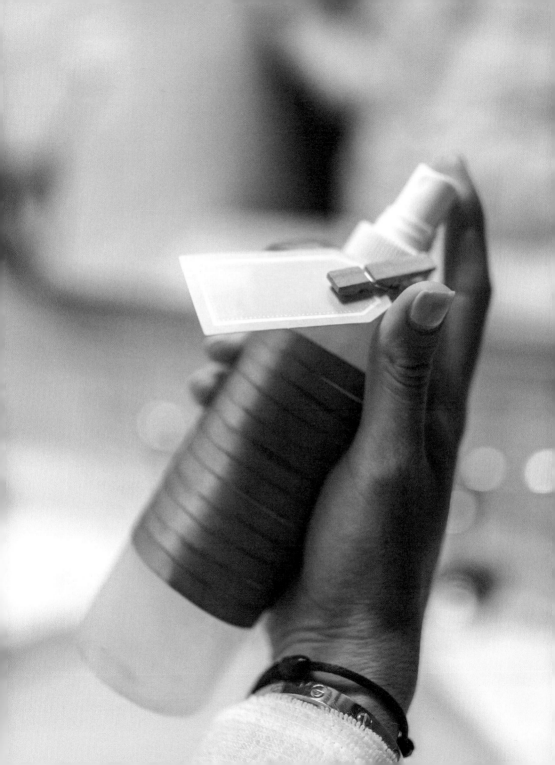

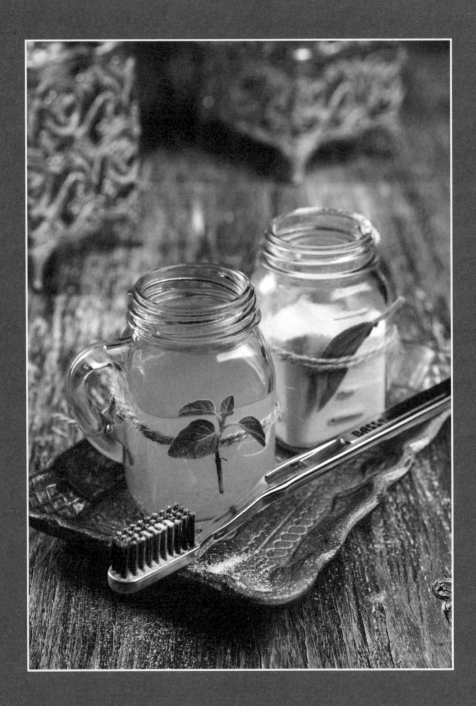

HEALTH AND HYGIENE

Struggling to find natural alternatives for your hygiene products that actually work as well as your commercial standbys full of synthetic ingredients? Look no further.

Sage and Sea Salt Whitening Tooth Powder
Holy Basil Mouth Rinse
Shaving Cream
Deodorant
Flu and Sinus Vapor Rub
Moisturizing Bug Repellent
After Sun Relief Spray

SAGE AND SEA SALT WHITENING TOOTH POWDER

Sage is a natural tooth whitener. Mixed with baking soda and salt, this powder will keep your whole mouth fresh and clean. A drop or two of peppermint extract will make the powder taste less salty.

MAKES I OUNCE

1 tablespoon dried sage
1 tablespoon baking soda
1 teaspoon sea salt
1 to 2 drops peppermint extract (optional)

Place the sage in a spice or coffee grinder and grind to a fine powder. Mix with the remaining ingredients in a small bowl and transfer to a lidded glass jar.

To use: Dip a damp toothbrush in a small dish of the prepared powder and massage your teeth and gums.

Store in its sealed glass jar in a cool, dark place. For maximum freshness and potency, please use within 6 months.

✦ ✦ ✦ ✦

APOTHECARY TIP

If you prefer to use a ready-made paste, add a tablespoon of coconut oil to the mixture.

✦ ✦ ✦ ✦

HOLY BASIL MOUTH RINSE

This effective rinse will kill bacteria, strengthen your gums, and keep your mouth fresh and clean.

MAKES I CUP

2 tablespoons dried holy basil (tulsi)
1 cup boiling water
1 tablespoon raw apple cider vinegar
1 teaspoon fresh lemon juice

Place the holy basil in a small bowl, pour the boiling water over the basil, and allow to steep for 15 minutes. Strain and allow to cool. Add the vinegar and lemon juice to the mixture and transfer to a lidded glass jar. Cover and shake.

To use: Rinse your mouth by swishing the mouthwash around for several minutes before spitting out. Use after brushing or whenever you need to refresh your mouth.

Store in its sealed glass jar in the refrigerator. For maximum freshness and potency, please use within 1 week.

+ + + +

APOTHECARY TIP

Parsley, mint, basil, and thyme all make effective ingredients for your own mouthwash variation.
These natural alternatives to your commercial toothpaste and mouthwash remove plaque, soothe your gums, and freshen your breath without damaging tooth enamel.

+ + + +

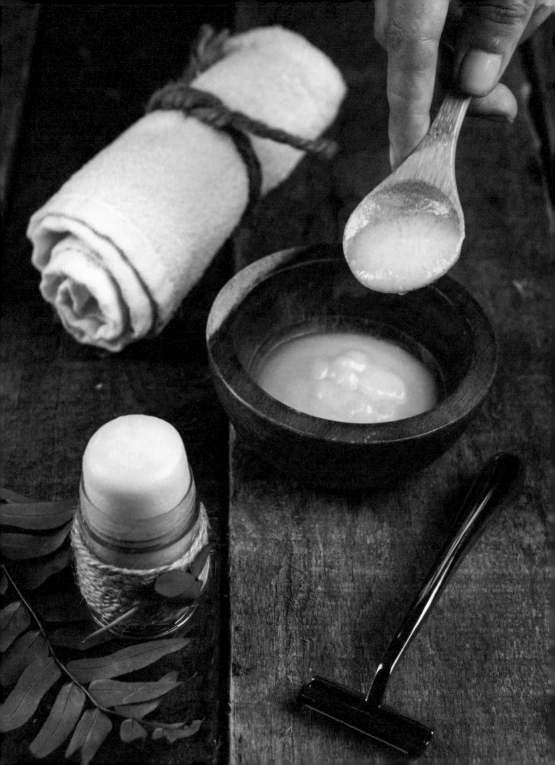

SHAVING CREAM

Help prevent razor burn and skin irritation with this healing aloe and nourishing coconut shaving solution for the softest, smoothest skin.

MAKES 6 OUNCES

¼ cup coconut oil
½ cup aloe vera gel
2 drops lavender essential oil (optional)
2 drops sweet orange essential oil (optional)

Melt the coconut oil in a double boiler or a heat-safe bowl perched over a saucepan of simmering water. Remove from the heat and stir in the aloe gel and essential oils, if using. Transfer to a lidded glass jar.

To use: Spread a thin layer of shaving cream on your skin and allow it to soften your hair follicles before shaving.

Store in its sealed glass jar in the refrigerator. For maximum freshness and potency, please use within 2 weeks.

DEODORANT

Here is a list of toxic ingredients found in most commercial deodorants and antiperspirants:

- **ALUMINUM**, a primary ingredient found in most commercial cosmetics, has been linked to breast cancer in women and increased risk of Alzheimer's disease.
- **PARABENS**, a synthetic preservative found in many personal care products, disrupts our delicate hormonal balance. Paraben exposure has also been linked to birth defects and organ toxicity.
- **PROPYLENE GLYCOL**, a petroleum-based material, can cause damage to the central nervous system, liver, and heart.
- **PHTHALATES** belong to another class of chemicals linked to a variety of health issues, including birth defects.
- **TRICLOSAN** is a chemical classified as a pesticide by the FDA and as a probable carcinogen by the Environmental Protection Agency.

Deodorant Detox

Sweating is a vital detox mechanism. To support this process and protect yourself from potentially toxic compounds, such as aluminum, synthetics, parabens, and artificial preservatives, choose a natural deodorant and note that it will take some time for your body to detox and adjust to the natural formula. Be patient; it is worth it for your long-term health.

Here is the recipe for an all-natural solution:

MAKES 3 OUNCES

2 ½ tablespoons coconut oil
1 heaped tablespoon vegetable wax
2 tablespoons arrowroot or tapioca flour
2 tablespoons baking soda
10 drops peppermint, lavender, or sage essential oil (optional)

Melt together the coconut oil and vegetable wax in a small saucepan over low heat, stirring continuously until melted. Remove from the heat and whisk in the arrowroot flour and baking soda. Add the essential oil, if using. Mix thoroughly but quickly, as mixture will start to thicken.

Pour into lidded glass or clean deodorant containers of your liking and allow to set without covering. Replace the lid when cooled and set.

To use: Use as you would any other deodorant.

Store in its sealed container(s) in a cool, dry place. For maximum freshness and potency, please use within 3 months.

✦ ✦ ✦ ✦

APOTHECARY TIP

Keep in mind that when choosing essential oils for your beauty recipes, some citrus oils are better avoided if you spend a lot of time in the sun. Photosensitivity, also known as phototoxicity, is a reaction to essential oils that could cause sunburn or skin irritation when exposed to the sun. Here are the citrus oils that are phototoxic:

Bergamot essential oil
Grapefruit essential oil
Bitter orange essential oil
Cold-pressed lemon essential oil
Cold-pressed lime essential oil

✦ ✦ ✦ ✦

FLU AND SINUS VAPOR RUB

This vapor rub contains antibacterial and antiviral properties that aid in the healing of dry, stuffy noses and sore throats. This recipe will also soothe your dry, winter skin.

MAKES 2 OUNCES

2 tablespoons grapeseed oil
1 tablespoon castor oil
2 teaspoons vegetable wax
5 drops eucalyptus essential oil
5 drops peppermint essential oil
5 drops lavender essential oil
5 drops grapefruit essential oil

Melt the grapeseed and castor oils and the wax in a double boiler or a small saucepan over low heat. Remove from the heat and stir in the essential oils. Slowly pour into a lidded glass jar. Gently stir the balm and allow to cool and set before closing the lid.

To use: Spread the balm under your nose and on your throat, chest, temples, and back to help relieve nasal congestion.

Store in its sealed glass jar in a dry, cool place. For maximum freshness and potency, please use within 6 months.

MOISTURIZING BUG REPELLENT

There are plenty of reasons to stay away from traditional insect repellents. Natural deterrents not only smell better, but they contain no toxic chemicals. Mixing and matching the essential oil combinations will deter mosquitoes much more effectively.

MAKES 6 OUNCES

¼ cup neem oil
¼ cup raw apple cider vinegar
¼ cup witch hazel
15 drops lemongrass essential oil
15 drops lavender essential oil
15 srops catnip essential oil

Mix all the ingredients together in a small bowl and transfer to a spray bottle.

Shake the bottle vigorously and allow the oil to synergize for 1 hour.

To use: Shake the bottle and apply the repellent to bare skin wherever you might need protection.

Store in its spray bottle in the refrigerator. For maximum freshness and potency, please use within 3 months.

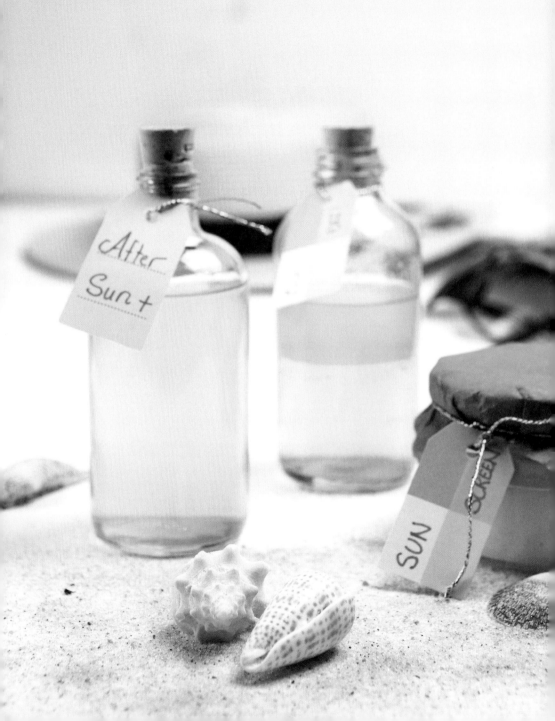

AFTER SUN RELIEF SPRAY

This chemical-free cooling spray is designed to help calm skin and reduce inflammation induced by over exposure to the sun.

MAKES 8 OUNCES

¾ cup distilled water
1 holy basil (tulsi) tea bag, or 1 teaspoon leaves
¼ cup aloe vera water
Juice of 1 lemon

Bring the water to a boil, then remove from the heat. Steep the tea bag or tea leaves in the water for 1 hour. Strain the infusion into a small bowl and add the aloe water and lemon juice. Stir together and transfer to a spray bottle.

To use: Shake well and spray onto your sunburned or wind-burned skin as often as necessary.

Store in its spray bottle in the refrigerator. For maximum freshness and potency, please use within 1 week.

Sun Care

The sun can help regulate sleep cycles, stimulate the body's production of vitamin D, and enhance general well-being. But if a little sun becomes too much, a whole slew of skin problems can occur—from premature skin aging and hyperpigmentation to skin cancer. Eating a diet rich in antioxidant compounds can reduce damaging effects and, when needed, choosing a mineral sunscreen with zinc oxide and titanium dioxide, instead of a chemical one, will create a physical barrier between your skin and the sun, blocking both UVA rays (which cause wrinkles and skin cancer) and UVB rays (responsible for sunburn).

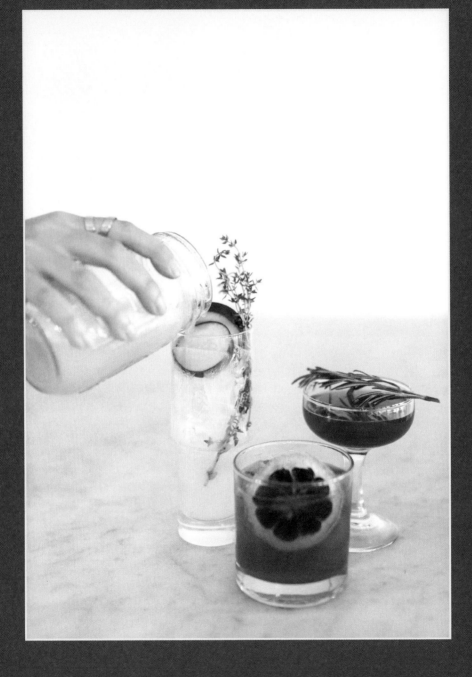

SPA DAY TREATS

The only thing more gratifying than a self-care ritual is a full day of blissed out beauty. Call the girls and take turns hosting a weekly spa day complete with sweet-smelling lotions and pampering potions. The following sips and snacks will keep you glowing from the inside out.

Cardamom Rose Chia Pudding

Mango and Pineapple Lassi

Pineapple Fire Cider

Agua de Sandia

Lemongrass Sparkler

Petals and Blooms Beauty Punch

Astragalus/Dandelion Spiced Chai

Magical Mushroom Hot Cacao

Thyme and Scallion Flatbread

Young Coconut Ceviche

Be Still My Beet-ing Heart Red Velvet Truffles

Mimosa Sorbet

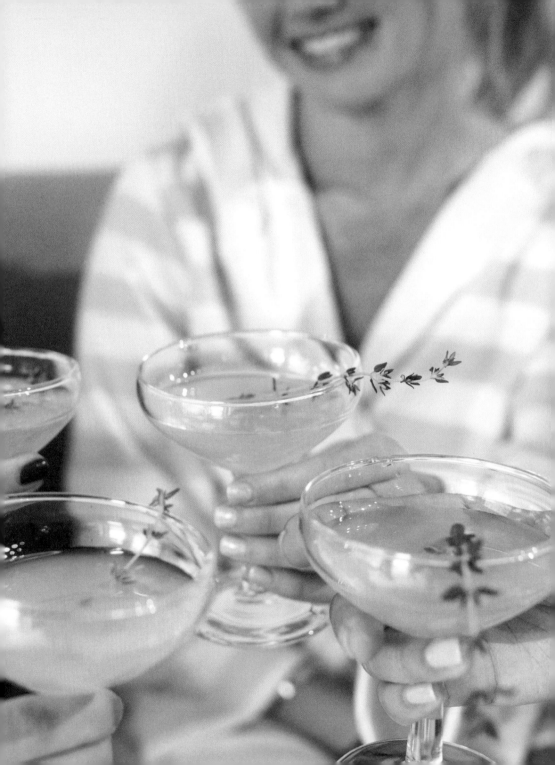

Spa Day Tips

For the perfect pampering beauty day at home:

- *Customize a pitcher of spa water with your favorite fruits and/or herbs*

- *Set the mood by burning incense diffusers, lighting candles, and turning on a mellow playlist.*

- *Ask your guests to arrive dressed in robes and flip-flops. Supply each with a stretchy headband and have fresh towels on hand.*

- *Create rotating stations: nail, foot, facial, massage, etc.*

- *Have plenty of snacks and drinks on hand.*

- *Have fun!*

CARDAMOM ROSE CHIA PUDDING

This lovely breakfast pudding packs in vitamins, minerals, and omega 3s that will keep you satiated without weighing you down. Chia seeds, in particular, contain powerful antioxidants that fight bloat and wrinkles, keeping your skin tight, smooth, and soft.

Prepare the pudding the night before, and you'll have a thick, creamy breakfast by morning.

MAKES 2½ CUPS

2 cups canned coconut milk

1 banana

3 tablespoons rose water

½ teaspoon ground cardamom

½ teaspoon pure vanilla extract

1 teaspoon maqui powder (optional)

Golden raisins (optional)

¼ cup chia seeds

¼ cup crushed pistachios

Combine the milk, banana, rose water, cardamom, vanilla, and maqui, if using, in a blender and process until smooth. Taste for sweetness and mix in raisins, if needed. Add the chia seeds and process briefly to combine. Pour the mixture into a bowl and refrigerate for 2 hours to allow the pudding to thicken. To serve, spoon the pudding into bowls and sprinkle generously with the crushed pistachios. Store in a sealed container in the refrigerator for up to 3 days.

BEAUTY FOOD SPOTLIGHT

Maqui berries are very rich in anthocyanins, which give the berry its beautiful purple hue. Blend 1 teaspoon of maqui berry powder for that extra-powerful antioxidant for beautiful, glowing skin.

◆ ◆ ◆ ◆

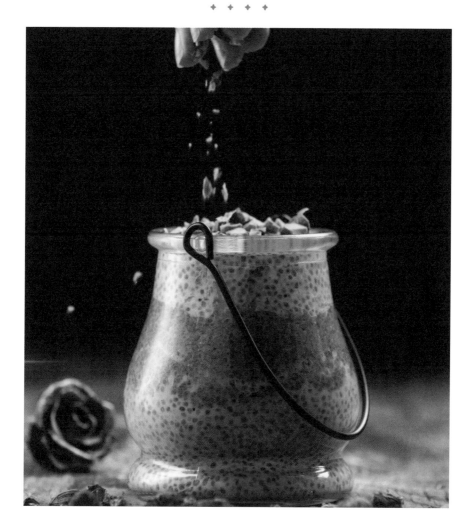

MANGO AND PINEAPPLE LASSI

A traditional Ayurvedic system-balancing drink made with yogurt, fruit, and spices, lassi can be enjoyed both sweet and savory. This golden tropical version combines the sweet goodness of mango and pineapple with the warming spices of ginger, turmeric, and cardamom, making this a truly cleansing beauty drink that supports gut health while eliminating bloat. Drink as is or add a frozen banana to turn it into a smoothie bowl.

SERVES I TO 2

½ cup chopped mango
½ cup chopped pineapple
1 teaspoon fresh lime juice
1 cup coconut yogurt
½ teaspoon pure vanilla extract
½ teaspoon ground cardamom
½ teaspoon ground turmeric
½ teaspoon ground ginger

Combine all the ingredients in a high-speed blender and blend until smooth. Serve chilled. Store in an airtight container in the refrigerator for up to 2 days.

✦ ✦ ✦ ✦

BEAUTY FOOD SPOTLIGHT

Both the mango and the pineapple in this delicious smoothie contain digestive enzymes that break down proteins and aid digestion. Mango is also an excellent blood builder, while the coconut nourishes the thyroid. Add the powerful anti-inflammatory compounds in the spices and you've got a true beauty tonic.

✦ ✦ ✦ ✦

Start the Day with a Beauty Tonic

Ease into your day with a morning ritual that involves drinking warm lemon water. Lemon juice delivers a collagen-building, antioxidant-packed vitamin C boost that supports detox and elimination essential to your glow. If you're feeling sluggish, feel free to stir in some grated fresh ginger or turmeric. Add a little freshly ground black pepper to enhance absorption or a pinch of cayenne to stimulate your metabolism.

For more energy-supporting, hormone-balancing and detoxing tonic ideas pick up my sister book, Zen and Tonic: Savory and Fresh Cocktails for the Enlightened Drinker.

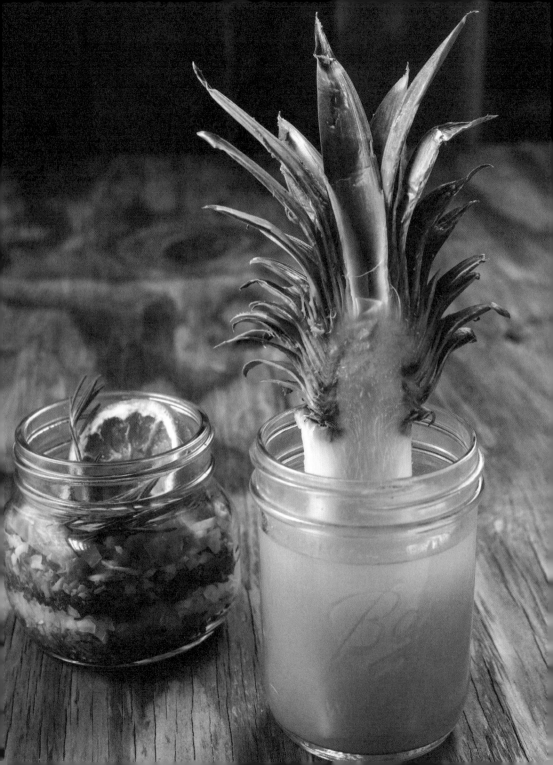

PINEAPPLE FIRE CIDER

Hot, pungent, sour, and sweet, the original fire cider was formulated by herbalist Rosemary Gladstar as an immunity tonic with powerful ingredients, such as horseradish, garlic, ginger, and hot peppers that kick-start your metabolism and support healthy weight loss.

I've adapted the original recipe to my own tastes here and encourage you to do the same.

MAKES 3 CUPS

½ cup grated fresh organic ginger
½ cup grated fresh organic horseradish
¼ cup peeled and finely chopped onion
¼ cup grated fresh organic turmeric
10 organic garlic cloves, peeled and finely chopped
2 organic habanero peppers, chopped
Several sprigs fresh or 2 tablespoons dried rosemary,
or 2 tablespoons of other dried herbs
Zest and juice of 1 lemon, lime, orange, or grapefruit
1 cup pineapple juice
2 cups organic raw apple cider vinegar
2 tablespoons pure maple syrup, or more to taste

Place all the roots, aromatics, herbs, and fruit zest and juice in a quart-size jar. Add the vinegar. Place a piece of natural parchment paper under the lid to keep the vinegar from touching the metal. Shake well. Store in a cool, dark place for a month and shake daily.

After 1 month, strain out the pulp, pouring the vinegar through cheesecloth into a clean jar. Be sure to squeeze as much of the liquid as you can from the pulp while straining. Then, add the maple syrup and stir to combine. Taste your cider and adjust the sweetness to taste.

AGUA DE SANDIA

This powerful take on the chia fresca, the natural energy drink, combines both watermelon and its rind for an exceptional nutritional refresher.

MAKES 2 CUPS

4 cups cubed organic watermelon, with rind
1 cup coconut water
¼ cup fresh lime juice
2 tablespoons basil seeds
Lime wedges, for serving

Juice, or blend, and strain the watermelon juice. Add the coconut water and lime juice and mix well to combine. Stir in the basil seeds and allow the mixture to synergize for 5 minutes. Pour into serving glasses and serve with a wedge of lime.

✦ ✦ ✦ ✦

BEAUTY FOOD SPOTLIGHT

This vibrant drink increases blood flow and your libido, thanks to the amino acid citrulline, concentrated in the rind. The gelatinous basil seeds, similar to chia in texture and flavor, cool the system and boost your metabolism.

✦ ✦ ✦ ✦

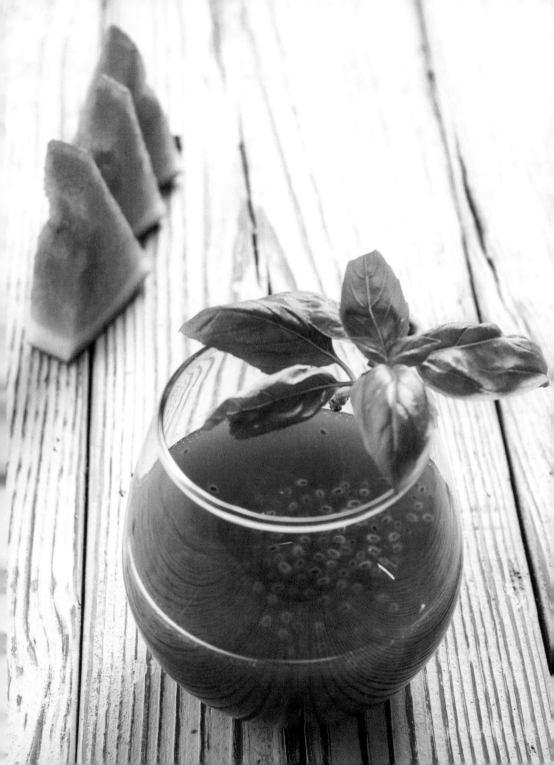

LEMONGRASS SPARKLER

This fragrant cooler, reminiscent of the tropics, is soothing and balancing. Aromatic lemongrass is chock-full of antibacterial, antifungal, and antimicrobial properties that keep skin glowing in all seasons.

MAKES 1 DRINK

LEMONGRASS SYRUP
MAKES 1 CUP

2 lemongrass stalks, sliced
¼ cup minced fresh basil
1 cup coconut sugar
1 cup filtered water

PER SPARKLER
2 tablespoons lemongrass syrup
2 tablespoons fresh lime juice
1 tablespoon fresh coconut milk
¼ cup sake
¼ cup sparkling water or probiotic coconut water

To make the lemongrass syrup:
Combine the water, lemongrass, basil, and coconut sugar in a saucepan over medium-high heat. Bring to a simmer and stir until the sugar fully dissolves. Remove from the heat and let steep for 15 minutes. Strain into a clean jar, cover, and keep refrigerated for up to 2 weeks.

To make the sparkler:
Combine all the sparkler ingredients, except the sparkling water, in an ice-filled shaker. Shake and strain into a glass with fresh ice. Top with sparkling water or with probiotic coconut water.

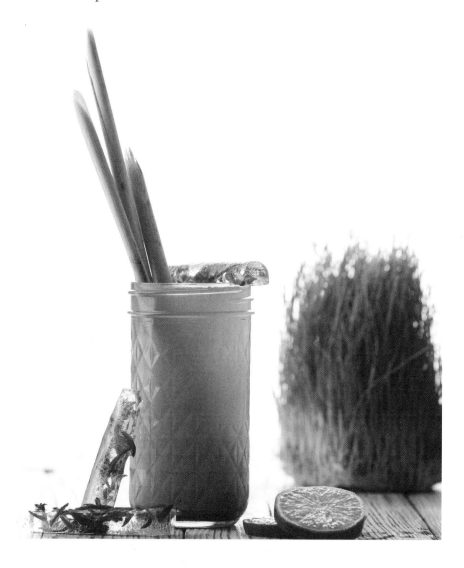

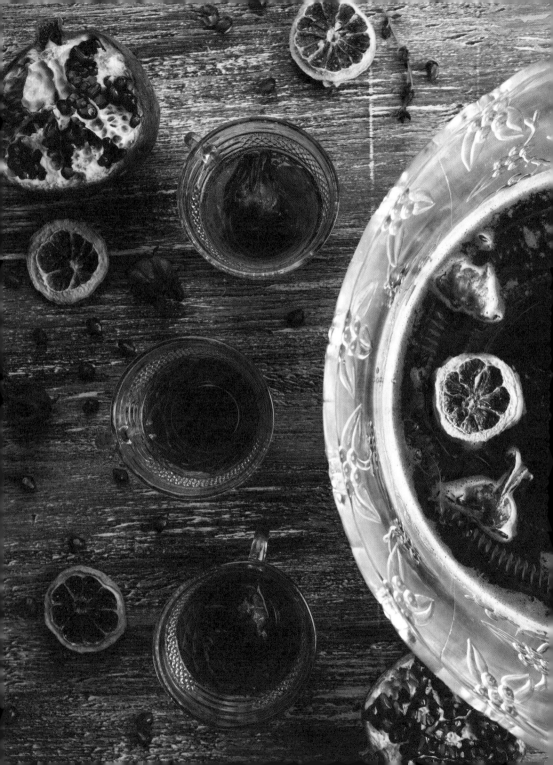

PETALS AND BLOOMS BEAUTY PUNCH

This bright, festive elixir—rich in the beautifying antioxidant polyphenol resveratrol—makes the ultimate beauty punch.

PETAL AND BLOOM SYRUP

MAKES 1 CUP

2 tablespoons culinary-grade dried rose petals
1 tablespoon culinary-grade dried lavender
2 tablespoons culinary-grade dried rosehips
2 tablespoons culinary-grade dried damiana (optional)
1 cup hulled organic strawberries
1 cup filtered water
1 cup coconut sugar

PUNCH

MAKES 8 TO 10 SERVINGS

1 cup Petal and Bloom Syrup
1 cup pomegranate juice
¼ cup orange blossom water
1 (750-ml) bottle rosé wine
1 (750-ml) bottle sparkling wine
Culinary-grade flowers and berries, for garnish

(continued)

To make the petal and bloom syrup:
Combine all the syrup ingredients in a saucepan over medium-high heat. Bring to a simmer and stir until the sugar fully dissolves. Remove from the heat and let steep for 15 minutes. Strain into a clean jar, cover, and keep refrigerated for up to 2 weeks.

To make the punch:
Combine all the punch ingredients, except the sparkling wine, in a punch bowl or pitcher and allow to synergize in the refrigerator for 1 hour. Add the sparkling wine before serving and garnish with colorful edible blooms and an assortment of berries.

❖ ❖ ❖ ❖

BEAUTY FOOD SPOTLIGHT

Indigenous to Mexico, the earthy damiana, with its figlike flavor, is an herb best known for its aphrodisiac properties. It works to uplift the spirits, relax the nervous system, and balance hormones.

❖ ❖ ❖ ❖

ASTRAGALUS/DANDELION SPICED CHAI

Your favorite chai blend gets a nutritional boost with this powerful herbal variation.

MAKES 2 CUPS

3 cups boiling water
1 cinnamon stick
1 tablespoon grated fresh ginger
1 tablespoon dried orange peel
2 cardamom pods
10 tongues astragalus root
2 tablespoons dried dandelion root
2 whole cloves
1 teaspoon black peppercorns
½ teaspoon echinacea root (optional)
Cashew milk, for serving

Place all the ingredients in a saucepan and simmer for 1 hour.

Strain and sweeten with coconut sugar or maple syrup to taste and top with fresh cashew milk.

✦ ✦ ✦ ✦

BEAUTY FOOD SPOTLIGHT

Earthy and slightly bitter, dandelions support the body's natural detoxification systems, balance hormones and blood sugar levels, and keep you looking trim. Astragalus, mild and sweet, also contains detoxifying properties that flush toxins and unwanted chemicals from your body.

✦ ✦ ✦ ✦

MAGICAL MUSHROOM HOT CACAO

Mushrooms are truly magical. They have long been used throughout Asia for medicinal purposes. There are at least 270 species of mushroom known to have various therapeutic properties. You can easily find a medicinal mushroom powdered blend to use or you can brew your own tea infusion. Please consult the resource guide at the end of the book.

MAKES 2 CUPS

Mushroom tea infusion
2 tablespoons dried chaga, reishi, or Cordycep mushrooms
1 cup filtered water

Mushroom hot cacao
2 teaspoons coconut oil
2 teaspoons pure maple syrup
2 tablespoons 100% raw cacao powder
1 tablespoon pure vanilla extract
1 cup brewed mushroom tea infusion
Pinch of sea salt or pink Himalayan salt
1 cup almond milk

To make the mushroom tea infusion:
Place the dried mushrooms and the water in a saucepan and simmer over low heat for 1 to 2 hours. Strain out mushrooms, keeping the tea.

To make the mushroom hot cacao:
Mix all the hot cacao ingredients in a high-speed blender for 1 to 2 minutes, until well blended. Serve warm and frothy.

BEAUTY FOOD SPOTLIGHT

With anti-inflammatory properties, mushrooms can help improve acne, rosacea, and eczema. They are also rich in vitamin D, selenium, and antioxidants that protect your skin against age spots, wrinkles, and discoloration.

✦ ✦ ✦ ✦

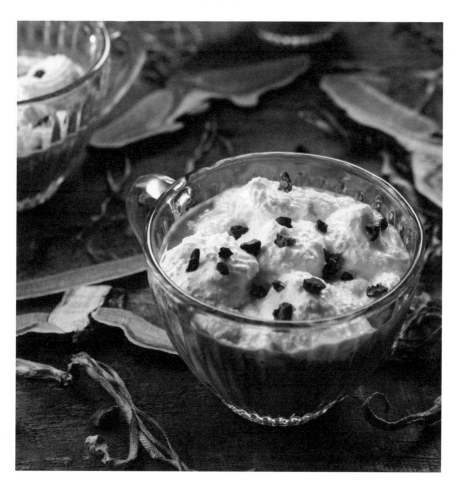

THYME AND SCALLION FLATBREAD

High in protein, essential fatty acids, and calcium, this unique, nutrient-rich flatbread is made with chickpeas as its base. Make it extra crispy to enjoy as is, try it with fresh arugula, peaches and cream cheese, or slather on your favorite sauce and fresh, vibrant toppings to make it your own.

SERVES 4

1 tablespoon coconut oil
3 tablespoons flaxseed meal
1½ cups cooked chickpeas, drained and rinsed
1 tablespoon raw sesame seeds
1 tablespoon fresh lemon juice
½ cup minced scallion
1 tablespoon dried thyme
Sea salt and freshly ground black pepper

Preheat the oven to 350°F. Line a baking sheet with parchment paper.

Place all the ingredients, including salt and pepper to taste, in a food processor and blend to create a smooth dough. Place the dough between two pieces of parchment paper and flatten, using a rolling pin. Place on the prepared baking sheet and continue to coax the dough into an even layer.

Bake until golden brown, about 40 minutes.

Remove from the oven and let cool. Keep in an airtight container for 3 to 4 days.

BEAUTY FOOD SPOTLIGHT

Chickpea flour is a high-protein, fiber-rich complex carbohydrate that can help stabilize your blood sugar and your hormones.

❖ ❖ ❖ ❖

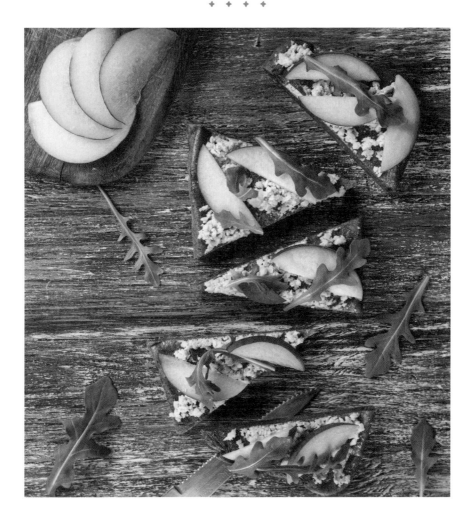

YOUNG COCONUT CEVICHE

A delicious riff on the traditional Peruvian dish of fresh seafood cured in citrus juices, this recipe uses fresh, young coconut as its base. The delicate coconut meat infused in citrus and spices tastes like the real deal.

MAKES 3½ CUPS

2 cups coconut meat (from 2 fresh medium coconuts)
Juice of 1 lemon, 1 lime, and 1 orange
1 orange bell pepper, seeded and finely chopped
1 yellow bell pepper, seeded and finely chopped
3 scallions, trimmed and finely sliced
1 red chile pepper, seeded and finely chopped
¼ cup fresh cilantro leaves
¼ cup fresh parsley leaves
1 teaspoon sea salt
Extra-virgin olive oil
Freshly ground black pepper

Scoop the coconut meat from the shells and rinse well. Keep the coconut water for drinking or to make Agua de Sandia (page 186). Cut the coconut flesh in small squares and transfer to a medium bowl. Add the citrus juices and toss to mix. Cover and set aside in the refrigerator for 30 minutes.

Add the bell peppers, scallions, chile pepper, cilantro, parsley, and sea salt and gently mix with the marinated coconut. Allow to marinate for another 30 minutes in the refrigerator.

To serve, divide the ceviche among serving bowls, drizzle with olive oil, and sprinkle with some black pepper.

✦ ✦ ✦ ✦

BEAUTY FOOD SPOTLIGHT

*Young coconut meat is an important source of potassium, sodium, and a
number of B vitamins, including folate. Its antioxidant properties slow
down the aging process by protecting the body from harmful free radicals.*

✦ ✦ ✦ ✦

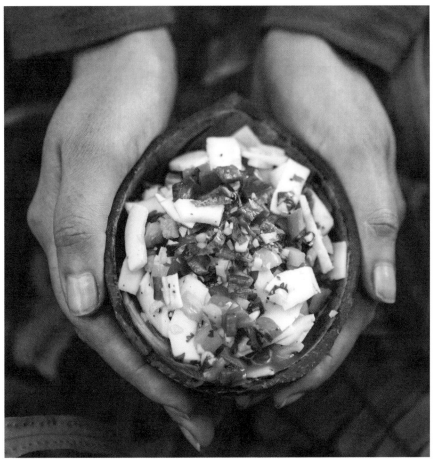

BE STILL MY BEET-ING HEART RED VELVET TRUFFLES

Despite the dark chocolate decadence, these delicious raw truffles are completely guilt-free. Made with antioxidant-rich raw cacao and energy-giving nuts and dates, they get their gorgeous crimson hue from their secret ingredient: the sweet, immune-boosting, and detoxing beet.

This homemade chocolate is made with just a few essential ingredients—virgin coconut oil, cacao powder, and pure maple syrup. The virgin coconut oil replaces the cocoa butter found in traditional chocolate, so while it needs to be kept in the freezer, it's a great way to sneak some coconut oil into your day. You can also use any toppings you'd like—dried fruit, nuts, and/or seeds all work lovely. These truffles melt much faster than regular chocolate, so be sure to keep chilled until ready to enjoy. I prefer them straight from the freezer.

MAKES ABOUT 16 TRUFFLES

TRUFFLES
1 cup raw cashews, soaked in water for 2 hours, then drained
8 pitted organic Medjool dates
½ cup shredded raw organic beet
1 tablespoon raw cacao powder
½ cup organic unsweetened shredded coconut

DIPPING CHOCOLATE
¼ cup raw cacao powder
¼ cup coconut oil
¼ cup pure maple syrup
½ teaspoon pure vanilla extract
Sea salt

(continued)

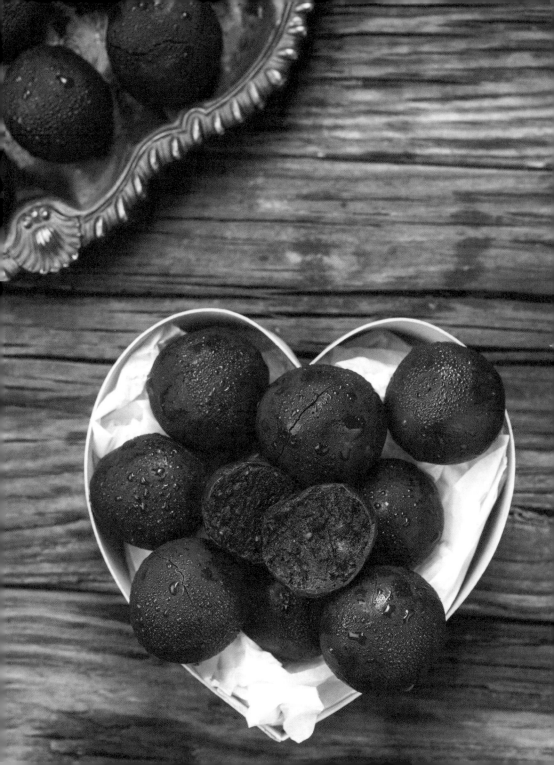

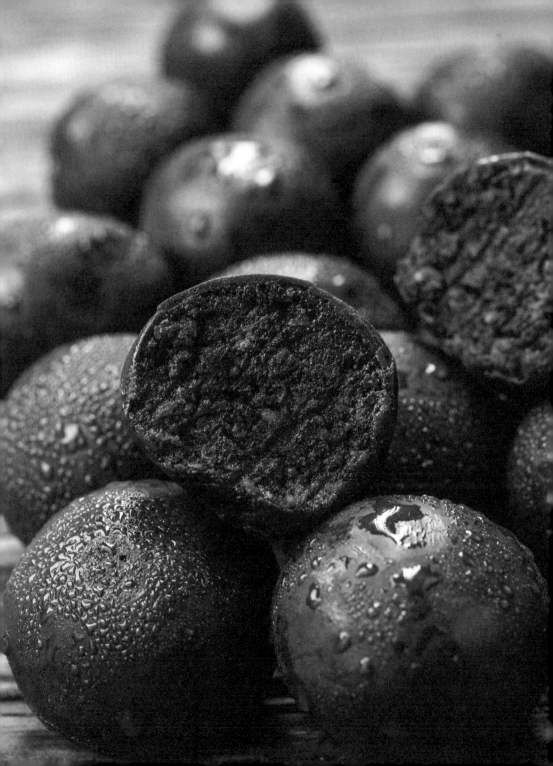

To make the truffles:

Place the soaked cashews in a food processor or blender and process until smooth. Add the dates and pulse again. Add the rest of the truffle ingredients and process into a smooth, moist dough.

Transfer the mixture to a bowl, cover, and place in the refrigerator for 30 minutes.

Remove from the refrigerator and hand roll to form balls. Place the balls on a plate and chill in the freezer for 30 minutes.

To make the dipping chocolate:

Place the coconut oil in a medium saucepan and melt over low heat. Remove from the heat and whisk in the cacao powder, maple syrup, and vanilla until smooth. Add a pinch of sea salt or to taste.

Remove the chilled truffle balls from the freezer. Insert a toothpick into each ball, dip a truffle into the molten chocolate, and remove from the chocolate. The chocolate will begin to solidify immediately. Working swiftly, give the ball a second dip for a thicker chocolate layer. Carefully remove the toothpick and place the truffle onto a large plate. Repeat with the remaining balls. Since this chocolate melts much faster than regular chocolate, store in the freezer until serving.

✦ ✦ ✦ ✦

BEAUTY FOOD SPOTLIGHT

With the highest concentration of antioxidants of any other food, cacao is a veritable beauty treat that promotes shiny hair, beautiful nails, and glowing skin. It also blocks the formation of wrinkles, thanks to the phytochemical epicatechin.

✦ ✦ ✦ ✦

MIMOSA SORBET

One mouthful of this refreshingly sparkling sorbet and you'll feel its detoxifying properties in action.

SERVES 6

6 oranges
¼ cup coconut sugar
½ cup water
1 cup champagne or sparkling wine
1 teaspoon orange blossom water (optional)
Fruit, for serving

Place a shallow glass dish in the freezer to chill for at least 30 minutes.

Cut the top off each orange and scoop out the pulp. Reserve the pulp for later use. Discard the tops and place the empty orange shells in the freezer to chill.

Muddle the orange pulp to remove as much juice as possible, adding additional juice, if necessary, to make 1½ cups.

Combine the water and sugar in a small saucepan and bring to a boil. When the sugar has dissolved, remove from the heat and allow to cool completely. Mix with the orange juice and champagne.

Pour the mixture into the chilled dish and place in the freezer for 2 to 3 hours, mixing gently with a fork every 20 minutes until it forms ice crystals and thickens. The frequent mixing will keep the sorbet from freezing into a solid block. Fill the orange shells with the frozen sorbet mixture and serve with fruit immediately.

KITCHEN NOTE

As an alternative, do it the Italian way, and turn your sorbet into a drink. Sgroppino, a slushy combination of sorbet, vodka, and prosecco, is commonly served in Italy as a palate cleanser, a dessert, or as a predinner drink.

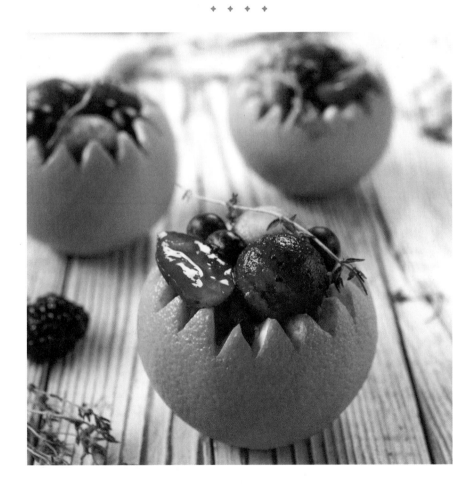

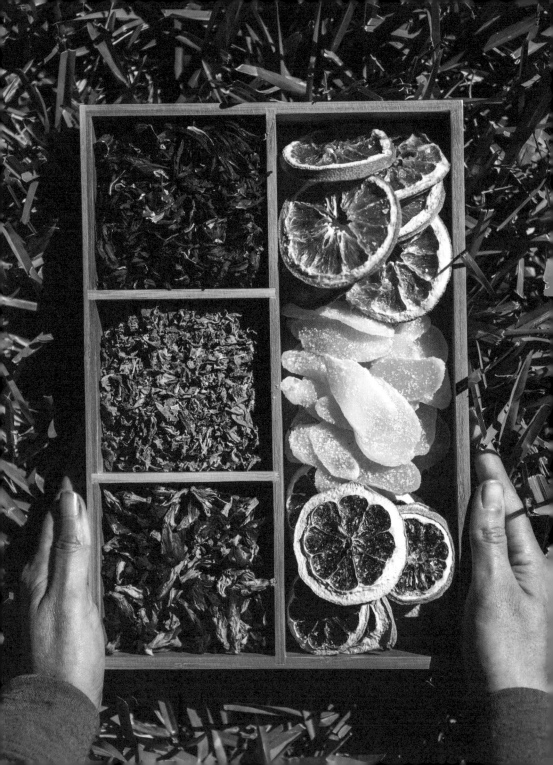

BASIC APOTHECARY TECHNIQUES

DECOCTIONS

Decoctions are simmered teas that are perfect for the extraction of hard roots, dried berries, barks, and seeds.

Place 3 tablespoons of dried herbs into a small saucepan.

Cover the herbs with a quart of cold water and slowly heat the water to a simmer.

Allow to simmer, covered, for 20 to 45 minutes, then strain.

HOT INFUSIONS

Hot infusions draw out vitamins, enzymes, and aromatic volatile oils from delicate parts of the plant, such as the leaves and flowers.

Using 1 to 3 tablespoons of dried herbs:

Pour hot water over the herbs and cover to keep the essential oils from escaping.

Allow to steep for 15 minutes to 1 hour, then strain.

INFUSED OILS

SUN INFUSION:

Use the sun to naturally infuse oil with the goodness of herbs.

Place the herbs or flower petals of choice in a clean, dry, quart-size lidded glass jar.

Fill the remaining space in the jar with the oil, making sure to cover herbs with the oil by at least 1 inch. If your herbs or flowers soak up all the oil, pour more oil on top to ensure that the herbs or flowers are well covered.

Stir well and cap the jar tightly.

Place the jar on a sunny and warm windowsill. Shake at least once a day.

After 2 to 3 weeks, strain the herbs or flowers from the oil through cheesecloth.

Pour the infused oil into lidded glass bottles and store, sealed, in a cool, dark place. The oil should keep for at least a year.

HEATED INFUSION:

Place the herbs or flowers in the top of a double boiler and cover by at least 1 inch with oil. Gently heat the double boiler over very low heat for 1 to 5 hours, topping up the water in the lower pot as necessary, taking care not to burn the herbs. The ideal temperature using this method is 90° to 110°F. (Alternatively, you can use a dehydrator or a yogurt maker to gently heat the herb or flower infusion.)

Turn off the heat and allow the pot to cool.

Strain the herbs or flowers from the oil through cheesecloth.

Pour the infused oil into lidded glass bottles. Store, sealed, in a cool, dark place. The oil should keep for at least a year.

HOW TO DO A SKIN-PATCH TEST

We all have different sensitivities to plants and oils. If you have very sensitive skin or are taking prescription medication, do a patch test before exposing larger areas of your body to a substance. Apply a small amount to the inner part of the forearm, then wait 24 hours. If the area shows any irritation under or around the patch, don't use the product.

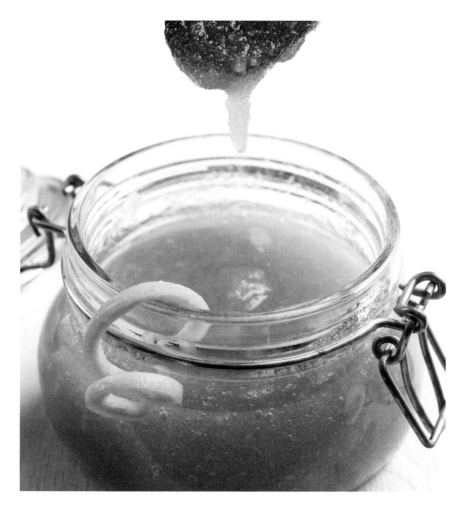

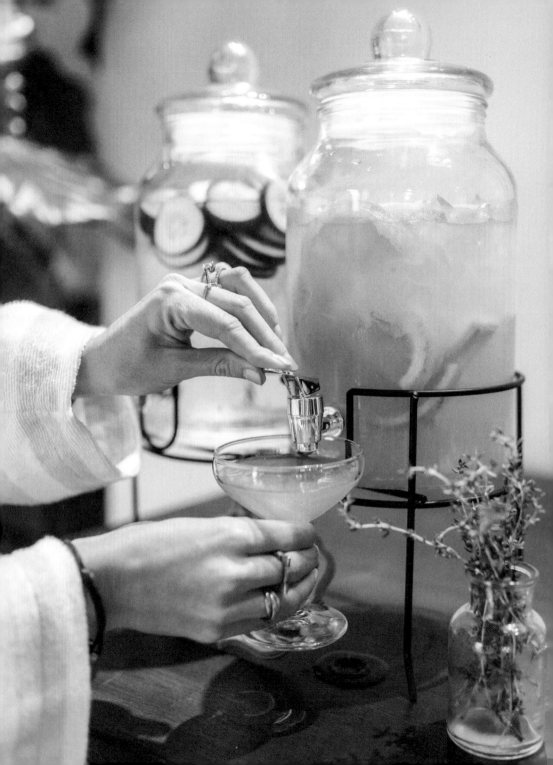

RESOURCES AND FURTHER READING

JulesAron.com: For the most up-to-date beauty and wellness news, recipes, products, and inspiration. Visit the site to arrange a personal consultation or to find out about workshops, wellness dinners, cooking classes, and online programs.

HERBS, SUPERFOODS, AND SUPPLEMENTS

Anima Mundi Herbals: herbs, elixirs, and tonics
Gaia Herbs: liquid herbal extracts
Herb Pharm: liquid, powdered, and topical herbs
Mountain Rose Herbs: herbs, spices, teas, and DIY supplies
Navitas Naturals: organic, nutrient-dense superfood powders. Quality source for your pomegranate, acai, matcha, and camu-camu powders
Root & Bones: quality extracts of adaptogenic herbs and medicinal mushrooms
Sun Potion: superfood, tonic herbs, algaes, and skin food powders
Urban Moonshine: herb extracts, tonics, and bitters

HOME BEAUTY-MAKING SUPPLIES

Aura Cacia: organic essential oils
Banyan Botanicals: organic bulk herbs and liquid extracts

Bramble Berry: soap and toiletry-making supplies

Bulk Apothecary: line of natural ingredients for toiletry making, including essential oils

Frontier Natural Products Co-op: organic and fair trade bulk herbs, spices, and teas

Liberty Natural Products: personal care DIY supplies, botanical ingredients, and essential oils

The Essential Oil Company: aromatherapy essential oil source

NATURAL BEAUTY PRODUCTS AND RETAILERS

Aubrey Organics: clean, hand-crafted natural beauty products

Bindi Ayurvedic Skin Care: Ayurvedic line of natural beauty products

CAP Beauty: beauty site sourcing all natural skin care, natural hair care, and natural makeup lines

Dr. Hauschka Skin Care: organic, holistic skin care with medicinal plants

EcoDiva Beauty: safe, eco-friendly, all-natural products for beauty and home

The Detox Market: beauty site sourcing green beauty, skin care, and natural makeup brands

INFORMATIONAL WEBSITES

Environmental Working Group's Cosmetics Database

Institute for Integrative Nutrition

Healing Spirits Herb Farm and Education Center

The Herbal Academy

Kynder.net

LearningHerbs.com

Personalized Lifestyle Medicine Institute

The Medicine Woman's Roots

The School of Natural Healing

Traditional Chinese Medicine World Foundation

FURTHER READING

Angier, Bradford, and David K. Foster. *Field Guide to Edible Wild Plants*, 2nd ed. Mechanicsburg, PA: Stackpole Books, 2008.

Aron, Jules. *Zen and Tonic: Savory and Fresh Cocktails for the Enlightened Drinker*. New York: The Countryman Press, 2016.

_____. *Nourish & Glow: Naturally Beautifying Foods and Elixirs*. New York: The Countryman Press, 2018.

Dugan, Ellen. *Garden Witch's Herbal: Green Magick, Herbalism & Spirituality*. Woodbury, MN: Llewellyn Publications, 2012.

Duke, James A., and Michael Castleman. *The Green Pharmacy: Anti-Aging Prescriptions*. Emmaus, PA: Rodale, 2001.

Drayer, Lisa. *The Beauty Diet: Looking Great Has Never Been So Delicious*. New York: McGraw-Hill, 2009.

Falconi, Dina. *Earthly Bodies & Heavenly Hair: Natural and Healthy Personal Care for Every Body*. Woodstock, NY: Ceres Press, 1998.

Gladstar, Rosemary. *Family Herbal: A Guide to Living Life with Energy, Health, and Vitality*. North Adams, MA: Storey Publishing, 2001.

Grove, Maria Noel. *Body into Balance: An Herbal Guide to Holistic Self-Care*. North Adams, MA: Storey Publishing, 2016.

Hart, Jolene. *Eat Pretty: Nutrition for Beauty, Inside and Out*. San Francisco: Chronicle Books, 2014.

Raichur, Pratima. *Absolute Beauty: Radiant Skin and Inner Harmony Through the Ancient Secrets of Ayurveda*. New York: Harper Collins, 1997.

Uliano, Sophie. *Do It Gorgeously: How to Make Less Toxic, Less Expensive, and More Beautiful Products*. New York: Hyperion, 2010.

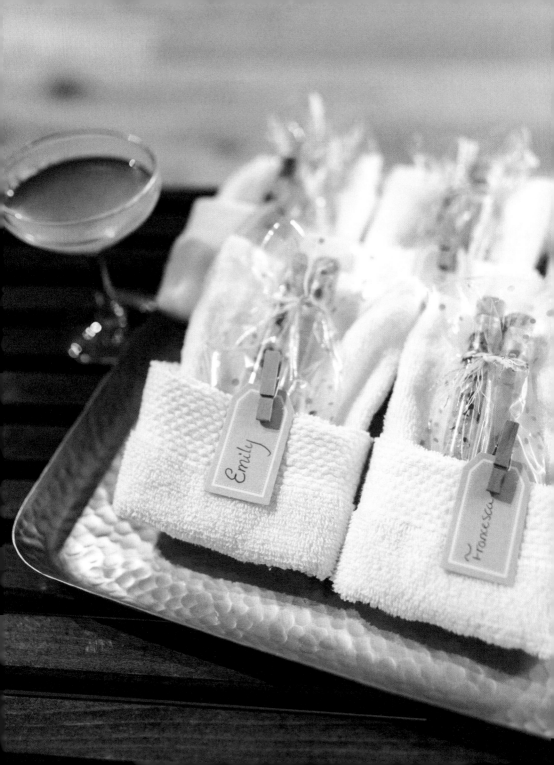

ACKNOWLEDGMENTS

The Pretty Zen collection marks my third and fourth books to date, and I am infinitely grateful for the tremendous opportunity to share these pages with so many of you beautiful souls. To the readers around the world who have been so passionately enjoying, supporting, and sharing my books, I thank you, first and foremost. May you find inspiration and guidance in these pages to fill your life with endless beauty.

It takes a group of masterful folks to produce beautiful books, and I have been lucky to have the same incredible team, give or take a few, throughout this journey.

Immeasurable gratitude:
To my literary agent, Marilyn Allen, always encouraging. Always supporting. Thank you, Marilyn, for believing in me. Your warmth and ongoing guidance mean everything to me.

To my editor extraordinaire, Ann Treistman, for your sharp and unwavering style. Thank you for your confidence in me and in my words.

To Gyorgy Papp, for making my recipes come alive with your photographs. Thank you for bringing my creative vision to life.

To Francesca Coviello, for working your magic with your sunlit lens. Thank you for adorning this book with your visual gems.

To The Countryman Press team, for the heaping spoonful of awesomeness poured into this book: Iris Bass for your thorough and capable care of my words; Aurora Bell for your unwavering grace and support; Steve Attardo, Devon Zahn, Anna Reich, and Jessica Murphy for your design and production talents; Jill Browning for your savvy marketing efforts. I am beyond grateful for all of your incredible talents. I thank you all for your time and effort.

A special shout out to the magical, creative hub that is the Social House, with all of its incredibly talented members—gracious, enthusiastic, and always willing to lend a hand—especially my lovely models, Emily Ravenna, Alina Dombrovska, Michelle Lara, and Megan Johnson.

And to my dear friends and family: Your tremendous support and amazing presence in my life is what makes this life a truly beautiful one. You are forever loved.

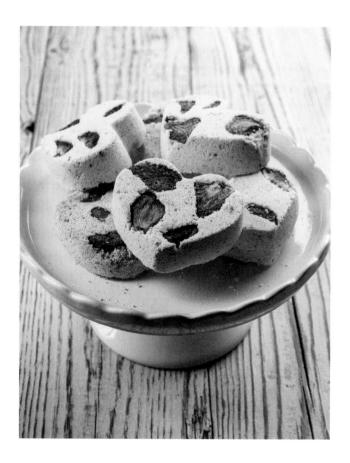

INDEX

A

Acai Berry Facial Mask, 46
activated charcoal, 85, 86, 120
After Sun Relief Spray, 175
Agua de Sandia, 186
almond meal, 114
almond milk, 65, 194
almond oil, 15, 26, 29, 40, 133
almonds, raw, 30
aloe, 124
aloe vera gel, 13, 43, 63, 67, 70, 71, 85, 86, 138,
     161, 162, 169
aloe vera juice, 60
aloe vera water, 122, 175
aluminum, 170
Apple and Green Tea Face Toner, 59
apricot kernel oil, 15, 27
argan oil, 15, 27, 155
arrowroot flour, 83, 112, 150, 171
Astragalus/Dandelion Spiced Chai, 193
avocado oil, 16, 27, 46, 65, 158
avocados, 13, 158

B

baking soda, 13, 98, 107, 110, 112–13, 139, 142,
     144, 166, 171
bananas, 46, 180, 182
base oils, 15–17
basic apothecary techniques, 207–8
basil, fresh, 188–89
basil seeds, 186
bath bombs, 110, 112–13
bath salts, 102–7
Beach Day Hair Spray, 162
Beauty Carrot Mask, 51
beauty tonic, 182–83

beet powder, 81, 83, 84
beets, raw organic, 200–203
bentonite clay, 32, 85
bergamot essential oil, 26, 59, 107, 108, 130,
     171
Be Still My Beet-ing Heart Red Velvet Truffles,
     200–203
bitter orange essential oil, 171
blackberries, 46
black pepper, ground, 183, 196, 198
black peppercorns, 128, 193
black tea leaves, 95, 114
blender, 17
Blueberry and Lavender Face Cleanser, 29
blush, 83
Body Care
     Caressing Calendula Bath Salts, 105
     Chai Exfoliating Lotion Bars, 114
     Chocolate Soufflé Body Butter, 127
     Cinnamon Ginger Sore Muscles Soak, 98
     Coffee Body Scrub, 117
     Detoxifying Charcoal Body Scrub, 120
     Dreamy Blue Bath Salts, 102
     dry brushing, 113
     elevate your bathing experience, 100–101
     essential oil properties, 108–9
     Herbal Rose Bath Salts, 104
     Jasmine-Tangerine Wash, 93
     Luscious Mango Body Polish, 119
     Luxurious Milky Bath, 96
     Orange Blossom and Lemon Balm Body
         Lotion, 124
     Perfume Balm, 130
     Personalized Bath Soaps, 90
     Rock Star Salts, 107
     Sea Mud Firming Body Wrap, 122

Body Care (*continued*)
   Sensual Massage Oil, 133
   Sleepy Time Herbal Tea Sachets, 99
   Strawberry Love Bath Bombs, 110
   Tea Time Body Cleansing Powder, 95
   Warming Vanilla Body Oil, 128
   You're the Bomb Aromatherapy Shower
      Tablets, 112–13
botanicals, dried, 90
brewed coffee grounds, 117
bronzer, 84

C

cacao powder, 78, 83, 84, 86, 127, 150, 194,
      200–203
calendula
   Blossom Shampoo, 149
   Caressing Calendula Bath Salts, 105
camu-camu powder, 43
cardamom, ground, 114, 180, 182
cardamom pods, 128, 193
Cardamom Rose Chia Pudding, 180
carrot juice, 51
carrot seed oil, 155, 160
cashew milk, 193
cashews, raw, 200–203
castile soap, 13, 93, 149
castor oil, 16, 35, 71, 77, 172
catnip essential oil, 173
cedarwood essential oil, 154
Chai Exfoliating Lotion Bars, 114
chamomile
   essential oil, 30, 99, 105, 108, 130, 149
   flowers, dried, 65, 99
   fresh, 36–37
   tea bags, 87
champagne, 204
charcoal powder, 120. *See also* activated
      charcoal
cheesecloth, 19
Chia Fresca. *See* Agua de Sandia
chia seeds, 114, 180
chickpea flour, 197
chickpeas, 196
Chocolate Lip Butter, 78
Chocolate Soufflé Body Butter, 127
chocolate truffles, 200–203
cilantro leaves, fresh, 198

cinnamon
   essential oil, 130
   Ginger Sore Muscles Soak, 98
   ground, 84, 98, 114, 117, 157
   stick, 193
citric acid, 110
citrus juices, 198
citrus oils, 59, 171
clay, 13, 32–33, 49, 51, 85, 95, 122, 144
cleansing
   DIY facial at home, 24–25
   with grains, 30
   with oil, 26–27
   powder, 95
   with steam, 35
   with witch hazel, 29
clove essential oil, 130
cloves, ground, 157
cloves, whole, 193
cocoa butter, 14, 78, 114, 127
coconut
   cream, 56
   meat, 198–99
   milk, 55, 96, 117, 180, 188
   oil, 16, 35, 38, 49, 55, 76, 78, 81, 86, 93,
      117, 127, 155, 157, 160, 162, 166, 169, 171,
      194, 196, 200–203
   sugar, 76, 119, 188–89, 191–92, 193, 204
   water, 67, 186, 188–89, 198
   yogurt, 182
Coffee Body Scrub, 117
coffee grinder, 17
Comfrey and Lemon Balm All-Purpose Healing
      Salve, 136–37
compress, 65
conditioner, 155
Cooling Eye Gel, 70
cranberry seed oil, 69
cucumber juice, 63
Cucumber Mint Aloe Face Wipes, 63
cucumber slices, 25, 70
culinary-grade flowers and berries, 191–92
Custom Blush, 83
Custom Sun-Kissed Bronzer, 84

D

damiana flower, dried, 191–92
dandelion root, dried, 193

Dead Sea salt, 102, 107
decoctions, 207
Deep Hair Conditioner, 155
Deep Pore Treatment, 35
Deodorant, 170–71
Detoxifying Charcoal Body Scrub, 120
Dipping Chocolate, 200–203
dirty list, 74–75
DIY facial at home, 24–25
Dreamy Blue Bath Salts, 102
dry brushing, 113
dry ground mustard, 142

E
echinacea root, 193
elevate your bathing experience, 100–101
elixirs, 40, 191–92
Epsom salts, 99, 105, 142
essential oils. See also specific essential oils
        overview, 14
        in perfume balm, 130
        properties of, 108–9
        in soaps, 90
eucalyptus essential oil, 108, 112, 142, 172
evening primrose, 27
exfoliation, 24, 46, 51, 52, 55, 56, 64, 76, 100,
        114, 137, 139
exotic perfume balm blend, 130
extra-virgin olive oil, 198
eye balm, 69
eyedroppers, 19
Eye-Friendly Mascara, 85
eye gel, 25, 70
eyeliner, 86
Eye Makeup Remover, 87

F
Facial Skin Care. See also cleansing
    Acai Berry Facial Mask, 46
    Apple and Green Tea Face Toner, 59
    Beauty Carrot Mask, 51
    Blueberry and Lavender Face Cleanser, 29
    clays, 32–33
    Cooling Eye Gel, 70
    Cucumber Mint Aloe Face Wipes, 63
    Deep Pore Treatment, 35
    Facial Massage 101, 44–45
    Facial Steam pH Balancer, 36

Grapefruit Vanilla Face Mist, 60
herbs for skin type, 37
Hibiscus Rejuvenating Cleansing Oil, 26–27
Ice Queen Beauty Therapy, 67
Lash Serum, 71
Matcha Cleansing Grains, 30
neck/décolletage, 64
Neck-Smoothing Compress, 65
Nourishing Eye Balm, 69
Papaya Face Scrub, 52
Piña Colada Face Polish, 55
Pomegranate and Rose Hip Whipped Mois-
        turizer, 38–39
Rose Oil Elixir, 40
Sea Siren Mask, 49
Strawberries and Cream Face Polish, 56
Vitamin C Love Serum, 43
Facial Steam pH Balancer, 36
fine-mesh strainer, 19
flaxseed meal, 196
flaxseeds, 30
Flu and Sinus Vapor Rub, 172
food processor, 17
foot powder, 144
formaldehyde, 74
fragrance, 74
freeze-dried strawberries, 107, 110
French green clay, 32, 49, 122
fruity perfume balm blend, 130
Fuller's Earth clay, 32
funnel, 19

G
garlic cloves, 185
ginger, fresh, 98, 128, 183, 185, 193
ginger, ground, 119, 182
glass jars, 19
glycerin, 17, 43, 85, 90, 93, 149, 161
goji berries, 56
Golden raisins, 180
grapefruit
        essential oil, 107, 130, 138, 171, 172
        juice, 60, 185
        peel, dried, 107
        Vanilla Face Mist, 60
        zest, 185
grapeseed oil, 16, 27, 90, 114, 119, 120, 130,
        172

green tea, 30, 67
green tea leaves, 59, 153

H
habanero peppers, 185
Hair Care
    Beach Day Hair Spray, 162
    Calendula Blossom Shampoo, 149
    Deep Hair Conditioner, 155
    Hair Frizz Tamer Spray, 161
    Herbal Hair Rinse, 153
    Mint and Avocado Hair Repair Mask, 158
    Natural Dry Shampoo, 150
    Pumpkin Spice and Molasses Scalp
        Treatment, 157
    Rosemary Hot Oil Treatment, 154
    Split End Healing Serum, 160
    when to wash, 151
hot oil treatment, 154
Hand and Foot Care
    Comfrey and Lemon Balm All-Purpose
        Healing Salve, 136–37
    Hand and Foot Scrub, 139
    Minty Fresh Foot Powder, 144
    Moisturizing Hand Sanitizer, 138
    Molasses Nail-Strengthening and
        Conditioning Soak, 141–42
    Mustard Foot Soak, 142
Health and Hygiene
    After Sun Relief Spray, 175
    Deodorant, 170–71
    Flu and Sinus Vapor Rub, 172
    Holy Basil Mouth Rinse, 167
    Moisturizing Bug Repellent, 173
    Sage and Sea Salt Whitening Tooth Pow-
        der, 166
    Shaving Cream, 169
heated infusion, 208
Herbal Hair Rinse, 153
Herbal Rose Bath Salts, 104
herbal water, 36
herbs for skin type, 37
hibiscus flowers, dried, 107
hibiscus-infused almond oil, 26
Hibiscus Rejuvenating Cleansing Face Oil,
    26–27
Himalayan pink salt, 104
holy basil (tulsi), 167, 175

Holy Basil Mouth Rinse, 167
honeysuckle flowers, dried, 107
horseradish, 185
hot infusions, 207
hot oil treatment, 154
how to give a great massage, 133
hydration, 11

I
Ice Queen Beauty Therapy, 67
infused oils, 208

J
jasmine essential oil, 93, 133
Jasmine-Tangerine Body Wash, 93
jasmine tea bags, 93
jojoba oil, 16

K
kaolin (white) clay, 30, 32, 51, 95, 144
kelp, powdered, 122

L
Lash Serum, 71
lavender
    buds, 95, 96, 99, 102
    dried, 191–92
    essential oil, 29, 99, 102, 107, 108, 112,
        138, 149, 169, 171, 172, 173
    water, 67
lemon(s)
    balm essential oil, 136–37
    Balm–Infused Olive Oil, 124, 136–37
    benefits, 14
    essential oil, 105, 108, 112, 144, 171
    juice, 43, 46, 77, 139, 141, 167, 175, 183,
        185, 196, 198
    zest, 119, 185
lemongrass essential oil, 173
Lemongrass Sparkler, 188–89
Lemongrass Syrup, 188–89
lime(s)
    essential oil, 171
    Lime in the Coconut Lip Scrub, 76
    juice, 76, 182, 185, 186, 188–89, 198
    zest, 185
lips
    Lip and Cheek Stain, 81

butter, 78
  scrub, 24, 76
  treatment, 77
lotion bars, 114
Luscious Mango Body Polish, 119
Luxurious Milky Bath, 96

M

macadamia oil, 16, 27
Magical Mushroom Hot Cacao, 194
makeup remover, 85, 87
Mango and Pineapple Lassi, 182
mango puree, 119
maple syrup, 14, 77, 185, 193, 194, 200–203
maqui berries, 181
maqui powder, 180
marjoram, 108
mascara, 85
masks
  body, 95
  facial, 25, 46–51
  hair, 158
massage oil, 133
Matcha Cleansing Grains, 30
matcha powder, 30
measuring cups, 19
meditation, 12
Medjool dates, 200–203
Mimosa Sorbet, 204
mindfulness, 12
Mint and Avocado Hair Repair Mask, 158
Minty Fresh Foot Powder, 144
mixing bowls, 19
moisture
  in natural ingredients, 13–15
  in oils, 15–17, 49, 69, 70, 117
  of skin, 10, 144
  Moisture-Rich Lip Treatment, 77
moisturizer
  body, 114, 127, 128
  facial, 25
  hair, 155, 158
  lip, 76, 78
  nails, 141
  Pomegranate and Rose Hip Whipped Moisturizer, 38
Moisturizing Bug Repellent, 173
Moisturizing Hand Sanitizer, 138

Molasses Nail-Strengthening and Conditioning
  Soak, 141, 145
Molasses Scalp Treatment, 157
mouth rinse, 167
movement, 11
Mushroom Hot Cacao, 194–95
Mushroom Tea Infusion, 194–95
mustard, dry ground, 142
Mustard Foot Soak, 142

N

Natural Dry Shampoo, 150
natural ingredients, 13–15
Natural Makeup
  Chocolate Lip Butter, 78
  Custom Blush, 83
  Custom Sun-Kissed Bronzer, 84
  Eye Makeup Remover, 87
  Lime in the Coconut Lip Scrub, 76
  Lip and Cheek Stain, 81
  Moisture-Rich Lip Treatment, 77
  Nontoxic Eyeliner, 86
  The Dirty List, 74–75
neck/décolletage, 64
Neck-Smoothing Compress, 65
neem oil, 16, 27, 160, 173
nettles, dried, 153
Nontoxic Eyeliner, 86
Nourishing Eye Balm, 69
nut grinder, 17
nutmeg powder, 84
nutmeg, ground, 157
nutrition, 11

O

oats, 14, 30, 95, 99, 150
oils. See also *specific essential oils*
  base, 15–17
  for skin type, 27
olive oil, 17, 52, 136–37, 154, 198
onion, 185
orange bell pepper, 198
orange(s)
  Blossom and Lemon Balm Body Lotion, 124
  blossom water, 124, 191–92, 204
  essential oil, 98, 130, 133, 169, 171
  juice, 185, 198
  peel, 96, 193

orange(s) (*continued*)
rind, 105
for Sorbet, 204
zest, 95, 185, 198

P
Papaya Face Scrub, 52
parabens, 74, 170
parsley, 167, 198
pea flowers, dried, 102
peppermint
dried, 144
essential oil, 63, 108, 144, 158, 171, 172
extract, 166
tea leaves, 158
Perfume Balm, 130
Personalized Botanical Soaps, 90
Petal and Bloom Syrup, 191–92
Petals and Blooms Beauty Punch, 191–92
phototoxic oils, 171
phthalates, 74, 170
Piña Colada Face Polish, 55
pineapple, 55, 182
Pineapple Fire Cider, 185
pineapple juice, 185
pistachios, 180
plant-based glycerin, 85
Pomegranate and Rose Hip Whipped
Moisturizer, 38–39
pomegranate juice, 191–92
pomegranate powder, 38–39
pretty Zen philosophy, 11–12
probiotic coconut water, 188–89, 198
propylene glycol, 74, 170
pumpkin puree, 157
Pumpkin Spice and Molasses Scalp Treatment,
157

R
raw apple cider vinegar, 14, 36, 59, 98, 153, 167,
173, 185
red chile pepper, 198
relationships, 12
rhassoul clay, 32
Rock Star Salts, 107
rolled oats, 14, 30, 95, 99, 150
rose essential oil, 40, 59, 69, 104, 109, 110,
130

rose hip oil, 17, 26, 27, 38
rose hips, dried, 104
rosehips, dried, 191–92
rose-infused almond oil, 40
rosemary
dried, 96, 102, 153, 154, 185
essential oil, 109, 112, 149, 154, 160
Hot Oil Treatment, 154
rosemary-infused olive oil, 154
Rose Oil Elixir, 40
rose petals, dried, 107, 191–92
rose water, 67, 161, 180
rosé wine, 191–92

S
sage
dried, 122, 166
essential oil, 102, 171
fresh, 36–37
Sage and Sea Salt Whitening Tooth Powder,
166
sake, 188–89
sandalwood oil, 109, 130
scallions, 196, 198
scalp treatment, 157
Sea Mud Firming Body Wrap, 122
sea salt, 14, 98, 102, 107, 120, 162, 166, 194,
196, 198, 200–203
Sea Siren Mask, 49
serum, 43, 71, 160
sesame oil, 27, 128, 139
sesame seeds, 196
Sgroppino, 205
shampoo, 149–151
Shaving Cream, 169
shea butter, 15, 69, 79, 81, 114, 136–37, 155
shower and bath treatments, 96
shower tablets, 112–13
shredded coconut, 55, 200–203
skin, 10
skin-patch test, 209
sleep, 11
Sleepy Time Herbal Tea Sachets, 99
snacks. *See* Spa Day Treats
soaks, 96–101, 141–42
soaps, botanical, 90
sodium lauryl sulfate (SLS), 74
spa day tips, 179

Spa Day Treats
  Agua de Sandia, 186
  Astragalus/Dandelion Spiced Chai, 193
  Be Still My Beet-ing Heart Red Velvet Truffles, 200–203
  body tonic, 183
  Cardamom Rose Chia Pudding, 180
  Lemongrass Sparkler, 188–89
  Magical Mushroom Hot Cacao, 194–95
  Mango and Pineapple Lassi, 182
  Mimosa Sorbet, 204–205
  Petals and Blooms Beauty Punch, 191–92
  Pineapple Fire Cider, 184
  Thyme and Scallion Flatbread, 196–97
  Young Coconut Ceviche, 198–99
sparkling water, 188–89
sparkling wine, 191–92, 204
spicy perfume balm blend, 130
spirulina powder, 49
Split End Healing Serum, 160
spoons, 19
steams, 24, 35, 36, 112–13
strawberries
  freeze-dried, 107
  hulled organic, 191–92
  Love Bath Bombs, 110
  Strawberries and Cream Face Polish, 56
sugar, 117, 119
sun infusion, 208
sunscreen, 75, 175
sweet almond oil, 133
sweet orange essential oil, 130, 133, 169
synthetic colors, 75

T
tangerine, 93
tapioca flour, 83, 84, 171
tea sachets, 99
Tea Time Body Cleansing Powder, 95
tea tree oil, 109, 120
thyme, dried, 104, 167, 196
thyme, fresh, 36

Thyme and Scallion Flatbread, 196
tips
  for healthy hands and feet, 145
  spa day tips, 179
toluene, 75
tools/tool kit, 17–19
tooth powder, 166
triclosan, 75, 170
Truffles, 200–203
tulsi (holy basil), 167, 175
turmeric, fresh, 183, 185
turmeric, ground, 51, 84, 142, 182

U
unsweetened shredded coconut, 200–203

V
vanilla bean, 128
vanilla extract, 60, 78, 114, 117, 120, 127, 130, 180, 182, 194, 200–203
vapor rub, 172
vegetable glycerin, 17, 43
vegetable wax, 15, 78, 85, 124, 130, 136–37, 171, 172
Vitamin C Love Serum, 43
vitamin E oil, 17, 26, 40, 69, 70, 71, 78, 136–37

W
Warming Vanilla Body Oil, 128
watermelon, 186
waterproof mascara, 85
wheat germ oil, 17, 27, 87
when to wash, 151
white (kaolin) clay, 30, 32, 51, 95, 144
witch hazel, 15, 29, 63, 87, 110, 138, 173

Y
yellow bell pepper, 198
ylang-ylang essential oil, 109, 130, 133
Young Coconut Ceviche, 198–99
You're the Bomb Aromatherapy Shower Tablets, 112–13

ABOUT THE AUTHOR

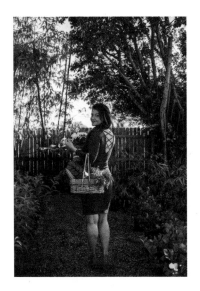

Jules Aron is a four-time best-selling author, holistic health and wellness coach, and green lifestyle expert. She is deeply passionate about a healthy, wholesome lifestyle that includes delicious, nutritious foods that fuel the body, mind, and spirit.

Jules holds a master's degree from New York University; received certification as a health and nutrition coach from the Institute of Integrative Nutrition; and is a certified yoga, qigong, and Traditional Chinese Medicine practitioner.

She is a sought-after wellness expert who has been featured in the *New York Post*, NBC News, TheTodayShow.com, *Thrive Magazine*, *Well + Good NYC*, and *Mind Body Green*. She is also a regular contributor to *Woman's World* magazine, as well as many other national media outlets.